Motivated to help and info authored an insightful autob sonal and revealing life chall forge a path toward understanding and healing not only for himself but undoubtedly for many others as well.

—Richard Hall, CEO

This book is an extremely informative yet heartfelt account of the author's struggle with thyroid disease. Clay has done a wonderful job of making this disease "human" for those suffering from the same or similar symptoms. By analyzing his own life's struggles and that of his family members, he teaches others how to recognize this medical condition in themselves. The reader is left with a sense of hope to cope with their own daily struggles.

—Gina Baresi-Spalla, Attorney

Clay's book is a witty, engaging, and ultimately inspiring account of a life filled with struggles, opportunities, fires, and misfires. It simply must be read by everyone who has ever said, "Why the heck did I do that?" or "What is wrong with me?"

—Pat Eubanks, Bank Vice President

This book is an outstanding autobiography that will help others understand the ever-increasing awareness of thyroid disease. It gives powerful personal experiences for people to relate to and understand this illness."

—Traci Kline, Teacher

# Why Am I Anxious?

One man's story of how not to
handle lifelong disease

# Why Am I Anxious?

## Clay Ballentine

TATE PUBLISHING & *Enterprises*

Published by Tate Publishing & Enterprises, LLC
127 E. Trade Center Terrace | Mustang, Oklahoma 73064 USA
1.888.361.9473 | www.tatepublishing.com

Tate Publishing is committed to excellence in the publishing industry. The company reflects the philosophy established by the founders, based on Psalm 68:11,
*"The Lord gave the word and great was the company of those who published it."*

Book design copyright © 2010 by Tate Publishing, LLC. All rights reserved.
*Cover design by Amber Gulilat*
*Interior design by Jeff Fisher*

Published in the United States of America

ISBN: 978-1-61566-571-6
1. Health & Fitness, Diseases, General
2. Biography & Autobiography, Medical
10.01.12

# Dedication

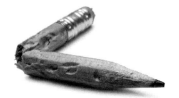

T his book is dedicated to my greatest gift in life, Abby. She has never ceased to believe in me, regardless and without question.

This book is also written in honor of my mother, Willa Lea, and my sister, Marcia, who never had a chance, in my opinion, to get their diseases correctly diagnosed prior to their deaths. It's also dedicated for all my blood family members I have left. All of whom I believe are affected by thyroid disease of one form or another.

To Tommy and Gina, Dan, Rox, Traci, Brad, Herman, Richard, Line, Simone, Pat, Tex, Terri, Doc Mike, and Jim; thanks for never giving up on me, regardless of how I acted or appeared at times. I hope it will ultimately prove to be the right decision for you for the rest of our lives. I can't imagine my life without any of you.

To the rest of you mentioned in the book by actual first names, I want you to know that I finally found the courage and guts to tell you the truth, if even by proxy. Now it's your chance to forgive me. I hope you all will.

The financial dedication of this book is to the National Thyroid Foundation, which Abby and I have just founded for children suspected of thyroid disease but who are unable to afford the laboratory testing. A great tree of practical love and sharing from a small acorn we've planted we hope will grow.

And finally, this book is dedicated to our Lord, who has chosen to save my miserable life at least three times for some purpose that my wife, friends, and I can only wonder at the miracle of. I hope this book was part of it and that you're happy with what I've done.

# Table of Contents

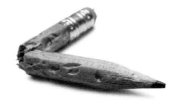

# Foreword

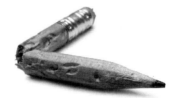

Clay Ballentine is my friend and patient of more than five years.

In *Why Am I Anxious?*, he vividly recounts the many obstacles he has endured and overcome since his early childhood.

He uses a simple and clear autobiographical style to examine these major life-changing experiences in some detail for us. Over time, he begins to question at length the relationship of his constantly recurring personal mood and physical issues to a possible influence of undiagnosed disease he hopes and fears is not mental illness.

The fact is, in Clay's case, it is thyroid disease.

In his very candid and straightforward narrative, I believe he sincerely hopes to motivate and assist the readers' interpretation and analysis of their own lives, behavioral, and health concerns—on a variety of fronts.

Anyone who is able to relate to his story could then follow a clearly outlined behavior path he has used to improve either their own lives and health, or the lives and health of their friends and/or loved ones.

I believe Clay wrote this book with the goal to help others—and I believe it will.

—Dr. Michael P. Vik, MD, P.A.
Austin, Texas

# Introduction

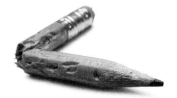

My name is Clay Ballentine, and I have thyroid disease. Specifically, two polyps, or benign tumors, one on each side of my thyroid gland. I have seen them in detailed living color through a sonogram, and it's obvious they are as old as I am. It is a birth defect.

I learned this fact at the tender age of fifty-one. It's my belief that most people aren't as bull-headed as I am and learn it by the time they're thirty-five or so in the incidence of similar birth defects. Thyroid disease is a difficult disease to diagnosis; the blood testing instruments to positively diagnose from blood samples weren't even made until about 1999. The early instruments struggled with accuracy and were quickly removed from the market. It's only since early 2002 that the instrument(s) were manufactured to provide physicians with a positive blood-test-based diagnosis when it wasn't an obvious tumor issue.

I would have had to have been much more honest than I ever was with myself, as well as my wife, family, friends and doctor(s), to have been diagnosed earlier than I was. I had way too much ego, false pride, and fear to admit that virtually any problems at all existed to anybody until I "blew up" and nearly died.

This is one of the greatest mistakes a disease-sufferer-in-hiding like I was makes. Ultimately, you wind up cheating only yourself out of what you so desperately need: love, prayer, and caring. And a good deal of medical help too.

The American Thyroid Association states that between 23 million and 47 million are at the clinical level of thyroid disease in America, or well more than one in ten of every group of folks you see. That's far more than heart disease and cancer combined. In my opinion, between thyroid disease and clinical anxiety, we have an epidemic in this country that is not even being discussed in the media, much less understood by most.

Since I have learned that I may have been hyperthyroid all my life and am now in a clinical thyroid disease situation, the only way I have found to relieve much of the anxiety and many of the side effects of my thyroid disease is by understanding—understanding both what is wrong with me as well as what has been wrong with me all of my life—and why.

Such understanding is a big part of the reason I wrote this book, because I thought if I could help you understand something about yourself, your health, or your behavior pattern(s) that seemed similar to some of the poor examples in my own life you'll read about inside, it might help you make the ultimate commitment to get a final and correct diagnosis, regardless of how many ugly truths you're forced to face up to.

Another intent of this book is to motivate you to take care of your own health and not to blindly trust any doctor or diagnosis without double checking (a second and/or third opinion if necessary) and then thinking about it an awful lot. The Internet is a free way to educate yourself, so I want you to take responsibility for your own health before any other issue in your life. This means you may need to sometimes strike out alone with a new physician or a different treatment option. I hope you'll remember something every good doctor I have ever had has told me: they conduct the *practice* of medicine. They know they aren't perfect any more than you or I are. Doctors make mistakes, miss things, and like any other detective, go down blind alleys in their investigations. I want you to always keep in mind that our health is *our* responsibility, just like our own happiness is too.

I don't want to throw stones at anybody, especially because there are so many dedicated and caring physicians like the one I personally enjoy. In fact, I should be the last person to throw stones at all. Instead of this book being titled like the popular series *Thyroid Disease for Dummies* or something like that, it should be titled more like *How to Have Thyroid Disease, By a Dummy*. That's a much more accurate title I must admit.

The book is written in autobiographical fashion because that's how an incurable lifelong disease evolves. Not because of any spectacular accomplishments or important autobiographical reasons on my part. The truth is, plenty have accomplished much more with as many or more handicaps than I've had - and started with less or nothing. The point of the book is not my personal autobiography or memoirs but the incidents of recognizing a growing disease that is first unknown and misunderstood, then hidden, feared, and covered up. Or perhaps, recognizing this in somebody you care for.

The result either way is simple: helping you find and deal with a disease or issue you may have or someone you love may have.

It's equally as bad, on both parties.

But it's not a death sentence, and we're not without hope. We can rebuild.

So I'll introduce this writing for those that want a true story about overcoming thyroid, metabolic, and hormonal type diseases, which can cause a devilish mixture of clinical anxiety, depression, and phobias of all kinds. These are many times combined with severe health issues like skin and bowel disorders, hair loss, weight gain and loss, sweating and temperature control problems, also including lost or low ability to concentrate, focus, and learn.

This is truly penned for you, the fellow sufferer of some of these disorders or friend of one because I haven't had a chance to tell you in person about all the mistakes I've made so that you might avoid some of them yourself.

It's my sincere desire that you'll find inside some laughs, some tears, and a few nasty truths you may relate to. But mostly it's been my foremost objective as I wrote to help discover what most of us are really seeking if we're sick or who have a close friend or family member who is sick—hope and answers.

Maybe more awareness all around about thyroid disease. Those of us who have this illness or give love and care to someone who does could sure use a bonus.

God bless and enjoy the truth down to the bone.

# Growing Up Hyper in a Hyper Home

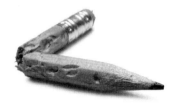

The three summers at Mrs. Shipp's house when I was four, five, and six years old were the greatest times of my life. Things hadn't gotten too bad at home yet, and getting in to Mrs. Shipp's house for three "mother's days out" a week was the same to every kid in this part of Dallas as being admitted on scholarship to Harvard.

Mrs. Shipp was the ultimate in love and affection. She had lost her husband some years ago, they told me, and had never remarried. She lived on a fantastic corner lot on the best street in the whole area in a blue-with-white-trim gingerbread house. It even had cedar shingles on the roof and cut cornice work along the entryways. It was always spotlessly clean, and whenever you entered the house, at whatever time, it always smelled like freshly baked sugar cookies.

We couldn't afford at that time for me to go there a full five days a week like I wanted to. But Mrs. Shipp still put my name on a plastic drinking cup along the windowsill for me to use just like I was a "regular" or full-time *"kid of mine,"* she would say. She also knew that I just wasn't like the rest of the kids.

She had seen me for my first two weeks there that first summer try to act like I was sleeping during nap time, which came each day between 1 and 3 p.m. I couldn't possibly sleep during the day, and it was torture to lay still in what she had converted from a master bedroom to the nap and bad weather playroom. Each child would have their own pallet of pillow and blanket to lie on, the regulars also having their name marked on their pillows in that laundry marker pen they used in the 1960s that smelled like gasoline. I had a name on my pillow too, but I couldn't use it any more than I could use a spaceship. I would wiggle, fidget, and stare at the walls and ceiling for two hours in torture every day while the kids around me slept and snored. But I figured I could take it; being at that amazing home was worth it.

Then one day, after she put all us kids in the nap room, she slipped in very quietly about twenty minutes into the nap time, just about the time every other kid was asleep, and got me.

We quietly slid out of the nap room together and closed the door. I didn't know what to expect, but she put her hands on her hips and looked at me very firmly and determined, like she always did when she wanted a straight answer from you and nothing but the truth. She asked me, "You can't take a nap, can you?" I simply told her, "No, Mrs. Shipp. I can't." We never discussed it again.

When nap time came the next day, there was no pillow and pallet laid out for me to sleep on like there had been each day before. Mrs. Shipp had something she needed me to do, she told the kids, while she physically held me back from the nap room. That immediately aroused the ire and jealously of every single other kid, but that didn't matter at all to me. All I could think of was that I was free of that charade and how horrible it was to listen to other people just sleep away while my legs wouldn't stop moving, much less my mind. I came to cherish the days I could spend at Mrs. Shipp's because she would never force me to nap, stop moving, playing, or sweating at her home for any reason and would never even comment on the "little differences," she called them once. At my home it was a little different matter, but that was okay; things weren't too bad there yet, and Mrs. Shipp's was always just a couple of days away.

Sometimes during nap time we'd have a cookie and watch *Guiding Light*, I think it was, or sometimes we'd play cards, particularly Crazy Eights. A lot of days, we worked on first and second grade school workbooks and all kinds of puzzle and math books, to give me an edge on the next school year, she'd say, but I know now she was desperately trying to use up of some of that extra mind energy I just always seemed to have. Besides, I never got tired of puzzles.

When I came back for the next summer, when I was five, she would let me go to the shop, an unbelievable privilege and one I kept secret from all the other kids as long as I could, especially the older ones who were, and had been, just dying to get in there. The "shop" was the only off-limits place for kids on Mrs. Shipp's entire property. It was Mr. Shipp's garage and workshop, and she had left it untouched after he died, until she gave me the key a couple of visits into that summer session. That meant I could go in whenever I wanted that summer.

The shop became my escape from the world, and I know now it was a really useful and educational time in my life as well. She had taken out any power tools, but this was 1962, and most people didn't have power tools; they had a "cranker," or a drill with which you bored holes in wood or metal by turning the wooden handle while applying pressure. Most all the tools a man like Mr. Shipp would have had would have been manual tools anyway, and the electrical fuse for the garage had been pulled. Very near the end of that summer, I had to rather sheepishly go to Mrs. Shipp at the end of the day, while my mom was waiting, and admit I had dulled every single drill Mr. Shipp had by working with them and drilling things all summer. She just smiled and kind of giggled then, big as you can imagine, reached over, gave me the sweetest kiss I've ever had, and simply said, "Don't worry, honey. I'll get them sharpened before next summer."

In the summer when I turned six, my third season at Mrs. Shipp's, she again gave me my own key for the shop on the first day. I had picked up a lot on my own and actually could now occasionally fix a thing or two around her house, especially the white picket fence that always busted in a couple of places where kids were always jumping it and the back door that got too much slamming. I was also allowed to run errands with *her* money for milk and ice cream she would run out of when she had a particularly full day of kids. This honor, one usually only given to a *nine-year-old* boy, was now mine, and mine at the age of six too! So now the younger kids began to want to hang out with me and want to follow me down to the store. I was becoming a "big man on campus" at Mrs. Shipp's house for sure. But my ability to keep my privilege of the shop, and my key, were lost very soon.

Two ten-year-old boys, the oldest children Mrs. Shipp would take (these were former regulars, and normally Mrs. Shipp did not keep children beyond the age of nine or do night or weekend babysitting), hid around the back side of the shop until I was just going in; then they jumped me.

I don't really remember the fight at all to be honest. My first recollection of what happened after they demanded the key and started to punch me when I wouldn't give it to them was the fact that I was still standing when the police arrived. One of the boys was down, and the other was gone. I know both my mom and dad came quickly and did a lot of talking to the police, and the one boy who was down was taken by ambulance to the hospital. I honestly don't think I had taken a hammer or tool against them because they jumped me just as I was trying to get in, but I couldn't tell anybody for sure at the time or today. I simply don't know what I did. But I can remember enough to know that the boy who was still down was hurt pretty badly, and I remember one of the officers repeating the phrase *"what a beating"* several times. I was really scared too. I thought I might be arrested, and I had never even been given a chance to say what had started it.

My mom took me out of Mrs. Shipp's right then; she said she was worried. I was a little bit worried too, but the worst thing of it all was seeing Mrs. Shipp's face through the rearview glass, forever etched in my mind as we drove off. She was afraid; she was upset, crying, very guilty, and unsettled too, but I was six years old now, and I knew what fear looked like. I got afraid too, but I wasn't going to show it to these people in the car with me.

•   •

Things started to go a little worse that summer after I was forced to spend seven days a week at home with my mother, even with my sister around (she was technically a half sister, but we never told anybody about that) to kind of act as a referee between us. But make no mistake; Mom wouldn't hesitate to turn on her either. Mom was very unhappy a lot of the time, jumpy, even more restless acting than I ever was, trembling with cold sometimes and then burning up. She had begun to get very moody, and the violence that would fly out of her was breeding a mistrust in me that lasted beyond her death. But it seemed sometimes she was just fine or just a little nervous.

I think I was just too young to make the connection that a lot of the things that made Mom seem crazy to us and those around us were really byproducts of her advanced but unknown and undiscovered thyroid disease. It's obvious when you're fifty-one years old and have the retrospect of time to see the similarities in our behavior that had already begun, but when you're six years old, you have a much tougher time figuring out what's happening. You get scared, your parents don't act like others, and you don't feel any love or security at home at all. This just exacerbates anxiety that is already above normal due to my unknown hyperthyroid disease. The same issues, like being unable to control my body temperature, irritability, venomous anger, and inability to sleep were the exact same issues my mom was having. Just in a smaller and younger version.

My sister, Marcia, was beginning to exhibit the opposite spectrum of my hyperthyroid condition, hypothyroidism. She had become quite moody herself, but I felt at the time it was in relation to Mom's constant attacks on us both. She wasn't angry nearly as much as I was or with anywhere near the ferocity, but she was depressed all the time and had begun to get quieter and quieter. This was especially bothersome as she had always been such a clown before. But now we would sit silently when alone for what seemed like hours at a time before I could get her to talk to me or laugh. She had begun to complain that she was unable to sleep too, but I didn't tell her that I hadn't been able to sleep worth a darn ever. In addition, she had gained a lot of weight quickly and with no reason. Her once perfect grades in school were falling as she approached graduation. She complained about how she could never concentrate or cram for finals anymore. Any modern doctor could look at the family unit and know in a second that thyroid disease might be an issue.

But in 1963, thyroid disease not been discovered. We had no chance then.

By now, my father had found and moved into an office apartment on the far side of town. It was true that his office was at least forty-five minutes away from our house in 1960s Dallas traffic, and he was a poster child workaholic. But, of course, the real reason was that the marriage was breaking down. I think both my sister and I were fooled for several months until the woman showed up with her "mother" at our house one very quiet summer afternoon on a Saturday we were all there. She was pregnant with my father's baby and wanted to know what my mother would pay to keep it all quiet. I only know they were quickly shown the door, and it was never discussed again.

From that day onward, not only did I have virtually no relationship or time with my dad, we also had no family for me to speak of in any manner. So I began what would be eighteen consecutive years of lying to close friends, schoolmates, and teachers as to why my parents were never present at any of my sporting events, parent/teacher meetings, parents' day, awards ceremonies, or anything. Frankly, I didn't want either of them there anyway.

Late in the summer of 1963, I was nearing first grade, as you could get in at six years old instead of seven *if* you were born before the first day of school that year, which in this case I can remember as being September 1 or some date like that. Wow, was I glad. I kind of felt like that birthday date of mine in August was like hitting the lottery. I wanted desperately to go to school. I loved books, learning, challenges, and especially recess; plus I didn't have to be around my parents.

But it had started to get worse and worse at home late that summer of 1963, and school hadn't started yet to get me out of the house. Mom was beginning to look quite a bit different. Her once beautiful, long, impossibly full, and thick jet-black hair had gone coarse, and it seemed like sometimes there were even some bald spots, but then they would fill in really quickly. I remember thinking, *This is impossible. I've never seen a bald woman,* but then it would go right away. Mom was a quite beautiful and striking woman when she was younger, doing both runway and trade show modeling and even doing mock-ups for the at-the-time famous Nardis house of fashion. But most days she was just not looking at all like herself, constantly complaining about her skin and looking quite a bit older, and she was unable to keep her weight up over 110 pounds, even though she was five feet ten inches tall.

A YMCA little league coach and super gentleman lived just across the street from us. He was known as "Coach K" for Koffendauffer. A bunch of us kids grew up playing ball in his yard, and he coached at the kids' portion of the giant set of ball fields that made up what everybody called the Y. One of the teams in his league was just flat out of players due to a couple of injuries. He knew I was only six, and the minimum age was seven, but told me, "That would be okay; let's just keep it down. You'll do fine." It was an unbelievable stroke of luck for me though and came at just the right time.

Now, I could go to the Y every day and practice baseball instead of being forced into staying home. So, just like a suburban office husband, every morning at 8 a.m., even though I was just six years old, I dressed in uniform, packed myself a sandwich, jumped on my bike, and headed to the Y—just like a job commute. It didn't matter that they wouldn't open the ball fields until about noon and the seven-year-old teams only practiced twice a week. I just wanted to get out of the house, and I could practice some even though the other kids weren't there yet or I had to work out with kids that were a good bit older. Most of the older kids were really great about it too, I have to admit; they just loved to play ball as much as I did I guess.

I did pretty well as a six-year-old in a seven-year-old league and kept my starting job at third base even when the kid who was hurt had come back, and his dad went into a rage at Coach K. Now, coaches from both the seven- and eight-year-old teams would start to use me as fill in whenever they had a need. *My gosh,* I thought, *this is heaven.*

School started just a few days after the end of the baseball season, and I loved it. I was away from home all day five days a week. It was really easy. Both Mrs. Shipp and my mom had tried to use of some of that excess "mind energy" by working with me using the same type of workbooks they were actually using in school. So it was no effort at all to have perfect grades; I'd already done the work the summer before.

One day right after President Kennedy was shot, I had to be a bit late home from school. I had become the first grade teacher's pet. Mrs. Ashmore was her name, and does anybody really forget that first grade teacher and/or not fall in love with her? She had asked me to help her with something for a whole class project, causing me to miss going home with the lady who carpooled my sister and me for a couple of years to and from school. Mrs. Ashmore even came outside to meet with the carpool lady who would always pick up my sister from high school right after me and take us both home, along with three other kids in a VW bus. She told our carpool mom not to worry, as I only lived less than one mile away, she knew perfectly where, and that she would drive me home when we were finished, in her car.

Only a few minutes more were needed to hang the posters and finish up anyway. It was no big deal at all, and the carpool lady sped off to pick up the middle and high school kids, who got out later, without a comment. Mrs. Ashmore even stopped us off on our way home at the Phillips Drug Store, a terrific traditional old-fashioned soda fountain and pharmacy. She treated us to chocolate malts. I held the door for her when we entered and left like my dad had taught me. I even waited for her to take her seat on the soda fountain stool before I sat. I remember feeling just like a stud on a date with a movie star. I'll never forget it.

I don't remember what caused it, if anything, what I said or didn't say, if anything, but I guess it doesn't matter. I just remember coming in the front door afterward, seeing my mom and starting to say, "Hi! Sorry I'm late," or something similar when I was knocked, feet flying over my head as if in some grotesque real-life cartoon, across the room and into the far wall of the living room, also crashing me against the side of the old Motorola phonograph that dominated that wall. It was at least twenty feet from where I'd been standing. I couldn't figure out what had hit me that hard, and I realize now I also had a concussion (the first of many I would obtain, but the only one my mom gave me), and then I remember being terrified that Mom had left the gas on the stove again only with the pilot unlit. We had just had a minor fire caused by that the previous week. That had to be it; our house had exploded! I couldn't get up at first, trying to rise then falling on the floor the first couple of times like a drunk idiot trying to rise up on ice skates the first time he's fallen.

I got my vision together and could see the drops of blood pooling on the floor beneath my head. There were two great things about that old house I grew up in: the incredible wood floors that were perfectly built with those sunken wooden pegs and the giant pecan tree guarding our front porch that I could never get my arms around even when I was seventeen. We used to have "twist and buff" parties with old blankets on those incredible floors, my sister, mom, and I buffing out the Johnson's Paste Wax with old blankets while dancing to Chubby Checker or something like that on the Motorola. You could easily slide for ten feet on those floors on a blanket just by barely pushing yourself with your hand. I remember thinking, *I'm in for it now; bleeding on these floors is a real no-no,* but I couldn't raise my head up enough to stop the blood drops. I was as dizzy as could be.

It hadn't been a gas explosion, a bomb, electrical charge, or anything like that. But what I did see when my eyes cleared and I could lift my head up was my mom still poised after the punch, totally frozen in her position like a odd statue, looking a bit like the famous picture taken a few years later of Mohammed Ali on the cover of *Sports Illustrated* after he knocked out Joe Frazier with the right cross tightly against the left shoulder. But the look on her face was not the same as Ali's expression of victory. It was one of grotesque horror, fear, guilt, and complete helplessness. I can still see it now as if it just happened a couple of hours ago.

I used my left sleeve to clean up as much of the blood off the floor as I could wipe up because my right arm seemed to have gone to sleep for some reason and wouldn't move right. By now, Mom was trying to talk to me, although she hadn't taken a step forward toward me. I didn't say anything to either her or my sister, who had somehow magically appeared and was looking on in complete terror. I headed to the bathroom to lock myself away from anybody and clean up.

I saw myself in our large double picture mirror, bleeding from both nostrils and from both ears, with a small cut over the top of my right eye (that was the stupid Motorola that caught me there, I thought). My left eye was closing shut, but I could still see out of it. I got an old towel out and used the ends to plug my nostrils and got a pair of Q-tips to plug up my ears and stop the bleeding. I then got another old towel to use to clean the blood off my face, neck, and shirt, but the shirt was ruined, so I was going to have to sneak another one out somehow. By now, my mom was beating insanely on the bathroom door—the hinges actually moving—crying, and screaming she would kill herself if I didn't open the door and talk to her. But I can tell you, Jesus Christ himself couldn't have gotten me to unlock that door.

I heard her fall to the floor in a very loud *clump* a few minutes later. It was loud enough to hear over the water running. I found out from my sister afterward that Mom had told her that she was having a heart attack and to call the ambulance; then she fainted. I also heard my sister calling my father at his "work house" and telling him what was going on with my mom medically but leaving out the part about the punch. She had pulled the long line of the phone near the bathroom so I could hear her conversation with Dad. He agreed to meet the ambulance people at the hospital. My sister was much older, had just turned seventeen, but only had a learner's permit to drive and was to stay with me until my dad got home.

I waited in the bathroom with the door locked until I heard the ambulance men arrive. I then pulled the Q-tips out of my ears and made sure my nose had stopped bleeding and slipped out of the bathroom while they were attending her. I knew where the suitcases were kept in the closet of the TV room. I got the smallest one out I could find very quietly in the dark, which was actually Mom's old cosmetic case. I didn't know or care; I just needed a suitcase, and I took it to my room at the back of the house while the ambulance men were loading my mom on the gurney to get her in the ambulance.

I still remember perfectly what I packed: my Bible, two Hardy Boys' mysteries, three pairs of socks and underwear, two pairs of nice pants, and two button-down collar shirts. There was some room left, so I added another Hardy Boy book and a heavy zip-up sweater. I closed the cosmetic case, and while they wheeled my mom out the front door of our house on the ambulance gurney, I slipped out the back door and down the alley where I would be unseen heading to the local bus stop.

Unfortunately, in that suburban part of Dallas where we lived, the buses didn't run past about 6:30 p.m. in 1963, and I didn't know that, nor did I know that by now it was well after 7 p.m. I was six years old. I didn't even own a watch. So I stood very quietly under and behind the tree next to the bus stop. The buses usually came about every hour or so that I could remember, and soon one would surely come by. I had over $5 saved up with me too. That would be plenty to help me find a new family even after the bus fare.

I heard the screaming for me from my sister just a few minutes later. She was screaming out the front yard then out the backyard for me to "Come home! Come home," and, "My God, where are you?" But from where I was waiting on the bus, she couldn't see me, and there was no way I was moving. When she went around the blind side of our house from the bus stop, which had to be less than a hundred feet from our front door, I crawled in the gutter at the corner because I knew she'd be coming up the street for me. I had left my bike on the back patio. She would know I had to be on foot because I never went far without my bike. But that cosmetic bag wouldn't fit down in the gutter with me! So when the street lights came on just a few minutes later, she immediately recognized the old blue cosmetic bag on the ground, and she eventually found me hiding in the gutter under the bus stop.

Nobody in my life loved me like my sister, Marcia. I knew that. So she slowly coaxed me out of the street gutter and promised me again and again, over and over, that she would protect me, warn me, not to worry, it was totally a once-in-a-lifetime event, and this could never happen again, especially with her watching for it all the time now. She admitted Mom had been having a hard time lately, what with all that was going on, and maybe she might be sick some too, but they just didn't know what from. But Mom really loved me and would never intentionally hurt me or my sister. But I knew the real truth: she couldn't even protect herself, much less me.

And all I really wanted in my life in November 1963 is out of that house; it was a crazy place.

We agreed right then, Marcia and I did, that we would never tell anybody what happened, and we just choked it down. Together.

As it turned out, there had been no heart attack either. My mom was diagnosed with a nervous disorder.

• •

Mom came home from the hospital with a full-time nurse. Marcia was too young to take care of her, and they thought it best to get a nurse to help administer the medications—tranquilizers and sleeping pills—for a while until Mom could handle it herself. This was especially true because my dad would never be there for her help either. For about two weeks after the incident, she was almost completely medicated into a stupor.

I can remember going in to see my mom with my sister a couple of days later, when the nurse had gone to the grocery store. She was completely sedated, unconscious, and lying flat on her back with her hands closed one over the other as if in prayer. I remember thinking at least she looked peaceful. I remember seeing the huge row of tranquilizers lined up in a metal dispenser across the top and the huge red sleeping pills lined up on the row below.

I looked at Marcia, and we both nodded at each other in the way siblings know and left. I vowed right there outside Mom's bedroom, in late November 1963, that you would never find me taking drugs like that to live. I would rather die.

           ●   ●

Y ou can't hide a hideous black eye(s), bump on your nose, and swollen face from all your neighbors and friends for long, especially during the school year; so eventually the rumors began to leak out. Pretty quickly, I found out that it didn't matter what my personality type really was or was going to be. I was becoming a loner simply due to the fact that many of the parents just didn't want their kids to associate with me now. I understood, and I don't blame them now and didn't blame them then either. Truth is ... I was a loner anyway.

I did still have three great friendships I had developed before school started that I could keep: Bill, H.L., and Ricky. We all planned to play football together on the official San Jacinto Elementary School team when we got to sixth grade, which at that time was the first grade it was allowed in public school. We made all kinds of plans for the future together like good kid buddies do. When we were together we also always acted like nothing like what had happened in the incident with my mom had ever happened. Just like it had been some kind of a bad dream that everybody had forgotten. Except, of course, they couldn't come to my house anymore. I had to meet them someplace neutral or go to their houses. But that was okay too; it beat not having any friends.

I found out another thing. There were two places where having crazy, separated parents and way too much energy didn't matter all that much: in the classroom when it came down to grades and performance and on the playing fields where it all came down to winning. So I went to work with everything I had to show these teachers, parents, and their kids they were making a serious mistake in acting as if I wasn't alive. By God, I would show them. In both places.

I made it through first grade with 100 percent one's, which were the highest grade given at the old grade schools; you didn't begin to get letter grades until middle school back then. I also had the highest number of Es, which were for excellence. No doubt being Mrs. Ashmore's pet kid helped a whole lot, but I could turn in my assignments as fast or faster every single day with perfect completion more than any other kid in class, partially because both Mrs. Shipp and my mom had had me working the workbooks and assignments at least a year in advance and partially because I was learning, just a bit now and then, how to really use my disease to turn on my mind and really go. It's pathetic really; at six I was already learning how to look smarter, play baseball better, or complete school assignments faster than most others, for my own benefit, mostly due to ego. I didn't understand how, why, or what was happening to me and couldn't regularly harness my disease, but I knew I was a bit different. Faster if you will, and more able to develop a fierce intensity and concentration at some times than other kids, and I would use the sickness when I could—sometimes on a conscious level, sometimes not.

Why is this different than trying to excel or just working harder than others? Rationalizations I was and would continue to use for years. I felt deep inside at that time, and today, that everybody enjoys watching a God-given talent perform at an awe-inspiring level, but those that cheat, for example by using steroids (in my mind, there's a similarity with excess adrenaline), are banned and ridiculed. I believe this type of behavior pattern is in reality the genesis of self-abuse, driven within a vicious cycle of disease, vanity, and denial.

Lump all these behavior issues that were developing, in my belief, to the ancillary side effects of the root problem of more and more anxiety caused by an unknown and undiagnosed disease. Anxiety continually grows unchecked if for no other reason than because your disease has not been discovered yet. But a disease doesn't care if it's been discovered or not; it's simply going to grow and worsen until treated or the body loses the fight. I can honestly tell you in my case I believe it wasn't full-blown self-abuse just yet. That would come later. Instead, most of the time I was still just trying to make the best of what I already knew was a bad situation and trying to meet what seemed like impossible demands of perfection from my parents.

My dad had begun to take me to his office with him every Saturday now to spend some time together. I always hoped that that was the reason he did it, but I have to be honest when I say both of us also knew it would keep my mom off of me for a full day. He didn't love me any or care much for me as a kid. I always wondered about that and why. It was years later when I learned I was born only four months after their marriage. So I finally got it. He had married my mom to keep me from being a bastard child. I could honestly respect that. I just couldn't understand it when I was so young. This was made even more confusing when they wouldn't tell me the truth of the matter.

He would take me to his business, which he owned and was growing in mobile home sales and reconstruction of repos, burnouts, and natural disasters. But we would reconstruct large buildings and offices too, after fires. I just was too young to hang out around those jobs, which were all over the United States. So he would have me clean up, pick up trash, chop the weeds, and put away loose tools around the Dallas complex in the morning; then, because I had "earned" my allowance that week, he would give me $2 to spend at the Bronco Bowl down the street on Fort Worth Avenue. And I could make two bucks go a long way on a Saturday afternoon in 1964.

Now, the Bronco Bowl was an entertainment nirvana famous around Dallas at the time. It had about a hundred bowling lanes, a slot car racetrack, a giant pinball arcade, and a huge pool table area in the center of the building with a snack bar and televisions all around. In the back, there was a huge indoor archery complex on one side, and on the other, my favorite part of the whole place and where I spent all my time: the batting cages.

There were four batting cages, and they didn't use the true hardball you use in baseball but that pretty hard rubber ball somewhere in size between a regular baseball and a softball. It was fantastic fun to hit balls there, and the four cages were clearly labeled outside, each one: "Little League—less than 50 mph," "Pony League—less than 70 mph," "Minor League—less than 85 mph," and finally my cage, "Major League—Warning! 100 mph." I would never bat in any of those "baby cages," even when I was just turning seven years old; it was always "Major League" for me.

Yeah, I missed a lot—especially at first.

But after a whole winter and early spring of coming every Saturday, George, the manager of the archery/batting cage area, and Newt, his assistant, began to let me pick up the balls and load the machines for them. They would then give me tokens, or what we called slugs, for free practice after I picked up. They had a big old manure shovel, and it didn't take me fifteen minutes to pick up every ball you could see and load the machines. There were two boxes for each machine: one for the regular load and a separate feeder, which could hold an overflow. George told me each machine, when you didn't "heap" it up on the separate feeder, would hold about five hundred balls, or more than a day's worth on a regular day.

He also showed me the control box for each machine's pitch control. Even in 1964, the batting machines were pretty good, and he showed me how to set the machine to just throw low curves, or high fastballs, or whatever I wanted rather than the normal random rotation I usually got. We even rigged a line that could reach all the way to the batting plate for me so I could use my foot to hit the switch, altering the style and manner of the pitches. George would adjust the arm each week so it would throw different types of curves and sliders at me too.

I was still missing some, but now I was hitting some too—and hitting some of them pretty darn hard.

Then another incident happened, and this time, it was just me.

It was only two weeks until baseball season began. The weather had been terrible, and two practices in a row had been canceled. I was going out of my skin with energy and anxiousness at this season's team. We were going to get Tye at pitcher, by far the best pitcher in the league, and my buddy H.L. was going to be at shortstop. If I could just handle the hot corner at third base and hit a lick, we had a great centerfielder already. I felt we were going to be bad, and I mean *really* bad. We all felt it, and we had all pasted skulls with crossbones on our batting helmets. But I needed some practice and energy burn terribly.

So one Saturday, just like usual, right at noontime, I asked George if I could just buy an hour or so on the machine for myself because I just wanted to hit. He said, "Forget it, kid; we won't have anybody in for a couple hours. Just go." So I rigged my usual line in the major league net, but after, I heaped up both boxes with every possible ball I could get in, including some from the other cages.

I began by calling pitches, low curves I could work on hitting to the opposite field, then hard inside sliders and fastballs that I would try to pull or just foul off; the big curves I was trying to learn to wait on so I didn't foul them off (George really had them set tough that week, I remember). I changed after a while, I remember, to hard fastballs, high and low, and I was really rocking then.

My goal was to drive the straight fastballs I got right back through the hole in the net where the ball came out of. I began to drive them right at the box. I changed again to low fastballs inside so I could bomb the homer-type swing you see the major leaguers do; then I switched back to the straight fastball, and the lottery shot happened. I busted a ball right through the hole and completely destroyed the pitching arm and a lot of the machine works too. It seemed like that entire Bronco Bowl went silent right then because it sounded like a bomb going off.

*Oh my God. That thing's got to cost a thousand dollars,* I thought.

I was absolutely on the verge of tears as I turned around to leave the cage to get George, and then I looked around. There were a bunch of people there, and I had never known it. My dad, for one; both George and Newt; about ten kids from an area high school team, who had been watching while waiting to hit in that cage too, still in their team uniforms from either a game or serious practice; their coaches, and just some folks from the bowling alley. I had no idea anybody at all had been there. It also didn't appear that there had been a single movement, sound, or reaction from any of them when the miracle shot I hit went straight back through the net to bust the machine, like they had been watching a while and expecting it. Not a single person moved or showed the slightest reaction; they were just looking at me.

It was George who spoke up first to break the pregnant pause, and he said, "That should be enough time now, kid, don't ya think?"

I said, "Sure, Mr. George. I'm awful sorry. I lost track of time; what time is it?"

He said it was about 3 p.m.

I had been hitting baseballs, constantly, with everything I had, one every eight to nine seconds nonstop, for three straight hours.

He had to be right because I saw my dad then and I hadn't called him on the bowling alley line they let me use to call him to come get me. I had forgotten to call, and he had come looking. I just couldn't believe how late it had gotten; in fact, I thought it was impossible. But it didn't matter anyway. I wanted to get away because I knew I had lost it a bit and was very embarrassed. But when I took that first step, my shoes were actually sloshing, completely soaking wet like I'd been standing in a puddle. I didn't wet my pants or anything like that. I was just completely covered in sweat, so much so that there was actually a puddle around the entire right-handed batting cage area, and it was my sweat that had done it. Later on, when I thought about it again, I could only imagine what I had looked like.

George bailed me out again after he saw me looking down at the floor. "It's that cooler actin' up again, kid. I'll get it wiped up." He sent Newt for the mop. And I sloshed my way out of the cage. But there wasn't any cooler anywhere near the batting cages; they were on the roof. Everybody knew that.

My father's look as I walked out of the nets was probably the most emotional look he had ever given me in my entire seven years as his son. But he just looked sad and totally puzzled. He should have been; he didn't know me one bit. But I knew that look from the high school kids as well. I had seen it before. They had respect all right, but they thought I was crazy too. Their coaches just looked concerned. I just wanted out.

We drove the entire forty-five minutes home in silence, a light sprinkling of rain steadily falling, the kind that causes you to mess with the windshield wiper all the time, especially on a 1964 car. Dad didn't know what to say. I didn't care if he did say anything.

When we arrived home, I stood up to him for the first time in my life and told him straight to his face, staring him in the eye as hard as I could. "Don't you ever tell Mom," I ordered. He simply said, "Okay, I won't. I promise."

I remember hopping up the steps to the house, all three of them at one jump, and opening the front door thinking, *God, I wish I didn't have to go in yet. I'm not even tired.*

• •

W e busted the league that next year. Coach K finally had his kids on his team; we were the Wolves. This was the group of us that had grown up all in the same neighborhood, in his backyard, playing whiffle ball since about three years old or so, and now he was our coach. We won sixteen straight games, eleven by mercy rule before the fourth inning. The championship game was called at the bottom of the third inning, fifteen to zero. Tye was absolutely untouchable all year, with a no-hitter and two one-hitters in games that both infielders would have told you they made clean errors on their part.

Late in the season, the pitchers started to only pitch me down and away, or force me to take a walk, so I had to begin to flush it to right field like I'd practiced so much that winter and early spring. Usually in little league, most coaches would generally put their worst field player in right field. So when I could tell they were going to pitch me that way, I would just close up my stance with my left shoulder turned hard in, and I would aim it right at the right fielder's head. I had more line drives turn into inside-the-park homers than should have been allowed by law.

There were few signs. We knew Coach K better than some of our family members. All he had to do was give us this look, and we knew whether to sacrifice, hit away, take, or most everything else.

Since I had been showing up at the fields early and accidentally ran into H.L. once, now almost all of us were starting to show up at the field just about every day around 9 a.m. Coach K noted this too, although he coached Pony League as well, which was a morning practice league. But he started coming by the Y fields almost every morning to work us out or give us four or five fielding drills to do all day.

Coach K had begun to notice my sweating problem.

He got me some Johnson & Johnson's athletic tape that made a sweat wristband before they were really invented. It stuck on me pretty good though, burning me badly when I peeled it off, so I asked Mom to let me tear up an old white bed sheet and use it under the tape. She said sure and actually helped me cut the strips. I would take a strip of an old sheet; cut it down; wrap it around my wrist, forearm, and just over the elbow; then wrap the Johnson & Johnson tape right over that (it also made it whiter, which looked really cool too). I also made a headband to wear under my cap (the sweat would just pour over my face at times, and Coach K said he was worried it would mess up my hitting).

The day at practice after I had worn them, Tye had two identical homemade sweat bands perfectly set up on his pitching arm and a headband tied on with some loose material hanging down like an Indian warrior (Tye was just one of those kids who was the coolest of all around, without ever trying to be).

By the first game against the team who were the favorites that year, we all had our homemade sweat bands on, tied up all over ourselves (some of them were kind of tied up a little loose with some dangling cloth so that they looked like those Apache armbands you've seen in the John Wayne movies. I swear!). Tye's dad had been a minor league pitcher in Tucson and had become Coach K's assistant when Tye moved up to authentic little league. He had real charcoal eye black like big league ball players would wear under their eyes (it's supposed to help with sun glare, but we just thought it looked cool—we played night games). He would put those black half moons under our eyes, growling at us while doing it to "toughen up" and "get mean." When combined with all that, some known neighborhood players, the best pitcher in the league, and ultimately those glued-on skulls and crossbones on our batting helmets, we were a real sight for them. They went out mercy rule in the third inning, fifteen to zero, and they really seemed relieved.

We were on a mission from God with Coach K, I'm telling you.

After the perfect season, Coach K wanted to have a banquet, but they had never really had one for baseball at the Y, so he organized it himself by selling advertising to the kids' parents. We had roast beef, mashed potatoes, and apple pie. Coach K had bought a bunch of trophies for all four age leagues: best pitcher (of course, Tye, in our age group), best outfielder, and best infielder (H.L. would win the next year, but Coach had to spread it around). I won League MVP.

The plastic trophy was about five inches tall with a figurine of a baseball player at bat. They had already put my name and stats on the trophy plate. It said, "W.C. Ballentine—1964 MVP," and on the second line it said, ".733 BA—19 HR." When I got that trophy, I almost passed out and could hardly shake the YMCA director's hand. I was sweating so bad and was so nervous I could hardly breathe (I swear the director wiped his hands off on his pants after we shook hands, but I didn't care; look at that trophy). Neither of my parents was there though. Mom was nervous and not feeling good that day, and Dad had to work again. Neither of them had gone to a single game that year.

They were both very proud of the little trophy I had earned after they got to see it. I got to place it in different spots of honor all over the house, like on top of the Motorola, the top of the TV in front of the rabbit-ears antennae, on the dining room mantel, all over. But the truth was that nobody else ever saw it because the fact was that nobody ever came over to our house. By now my mom's sporadic and inexplicable bursts of insane anger had caused not only the parents of every friend I had but also every neighbor within eyeshot to either avoid or flatly refuse to come to our home. It was okay though; almost all of them made me very welcome at their homes. That was good enough.

They broke up the team the next year, at what I heard was the loudest little league meeting at the Y ever.

Coach K, as director, had decided to move up to eight-year-olds; it was his privilege, so he could stay with us. He got to keep three of us kids—Tye, H.L., and me—but we lost every other player to other teams. We were absolutely devastated and went together to Coach K and said if our friends couldn't play with us, we weren't going to play with the Y. He looked at us pretty sternly; in fact, he got mad, and he told us, "What are you? Babies? Get your butts out to practice, and I mean right now!" That was the end of that.

We had no team around us but made the championship game after an incredible playoff with the second place team we were tied with, winding up with a twelve to five record. We lost the championship game in the third extra inning on a highly disputed call. When Tye, H.L., and I started the season and saw who we were playing with as teammates, we had just hoped to finish better than .500. To get in the championship game, win or lose, was a huge bonus we thought impossible. After the incorrect call was made at home plate, the game decided, Tye, H.L., and I just looked at each other, smiled, shrugged our shoulders, and then headed for the parking lot together because Tye's dad always took us home. I wouldn't even bring this whole thing up except for two rather important things:

1. It was the first sporting event my dad had ever come to see me play, and we had lost, despite the fact I tripled in our only two runs in the first inning and was intentionally walked six times after.

2. It was supposedly the biggest fight ever recorded in the Pleasant Grove suburb of Dallas after the game. The police were called because the parents got into it so bad after the referee's call and ensuing argument. I sure wished we had seen it, but Tye, H.L.,

and I were already in the parking lot when it broke out, more than a half mile away. Been around little league parents much? Don't call children immature.

Losing at team sports never gave me anxiety; it was a completely different set of feelings and emotions than failing your parents or losing in a solo sport effort like golf. If one gives everything they had to give in a baseball or football game and lost, the whole team lost. It's not a personal loss. It's obviously different in relationships and solo sports. Look at how high-profile professional golfers and tennis players take it personally, and some go through long periods of time without being competitive or winning, especially after an important loss or long losing streak. I think there are similar emotional feelings when someone has anxiety issues. Sufferers can seem to feel an awful lot like they're standing alone in front of a large crowd after an important loss. A lot of the time, this leads to another nemesis those of us with thyroid disease experience—depression. It doesn't take an awful lot of real or imagined "big losses" in a life to begin to get someone clinically depressed.

Need evidence? Just look at the growth of sports psychologists' use by sports professionals over the past few years.

We were all kind of the same emotionally about the loss, despite how the parents acted. But none of us needed a sports psychologist to explain why we lost, as we knew what kind of team we really had; we had given everything we had all season in every game, and it was over. We were second place, and that was pretty darn good this year—we knew it. Done. Let's go to Baskin-Robbins.

Coach K had an incredible banquet that year, and head football coach of the Dallas Cowboys, Tom Landry, was there as guest speaker. He spoke for about fifteen minutes and then handed out that year's awards to each kid. Unbelievably, because the level of play was really improving, I won MVP again. I was really trembling when I went up to get the plaque, and Coach Landry said something really nice. I know he did. I just can't remember because my heart was thumping so.

This time the trophies were beautiful wooden plaques. They had a picture of each kid on the bottom and a real metal plate with the accomplishment and statistic(s) engraved. Mine said, "W.C. Ballentine—1965 MVP," and on the second line it said, ".689 BA—15 HR." Coach K had gone to the Western Auto store, which was the closest thing we had to a sporting goods store in that part of Dallas, and bought five different sizes of pro-type black with two white stripes on the side baseball cleats with his own money. He had every single kid wear them in their team picture (all of us swapping shoes between each picture, cracking up with laughter at shoes two or three sizes too big or small) with brand new color-coordinated stirrups to wear up over the ankles. We looked just like pros in those photos down on one knee holding our bats. They were just unbelievable plaques for eight-year-old kids. The rest of the evening, I simply couldn't take my eyes off of it.

On the way home, my dad had been quiet at first, but it was a short drive to drop me off. Right as we were coming in our driveway, he pulled up short, put the car in park, but left it running.

He turned and said to me, "Hey, that wasn't that great a year this year; do you really think that was the best you can do?" I was a little shocked and stunned at first. I sort of thought he was joking with me, but he had never joked with me or smiled much around me in my entire life. I could see through the half-moon light of the T-Bird's dashboard that he was dead serious and beginning to look mad. I started to explain that the kid pitching that night was pretty good—and he only gave me one pitch to hit, which I tripled—but he cut me off sharply before I finished. "Sounds like excuses to me about sorry performance; your numbers are way down. Get 'em up next year; hear me?"

I just got out of the car as quietly as I could, said, "Yes, sir," and closed the car door.

Mom was almost unconscious from the combination of tranquilizers and sleeping pills she was taking by the time I came in the house. I had hidden the trophy under my suit coat to surprise her with, but from the sound of her voice welcoming me in, I could tell she would be comatose in minutes. She asked me in the most lucid voice she could muster up, "How did it go, honey?" I told her we had a great time and that Coach Landry was the speaker. I hid the plaque under the sofa before I went into her bedroom, so she never saw it or would know of it. I tried to talk to her some that night, like I hadn't been able to do in a long time since the incident, and she really tried to talk to me too—despite the devastating effect of all the drugs she was on. But the drugs won out. In midsentence with me, about five minutes into our first real conversation in several years, she passed out cold.

I waited about twenty minutes to make sure she was fully out. I grabbed up last year's little trophy, this year's plaque, and slid out the back door to the alley where the trash cans were. I buried both trophies deep in the fullest can, inside a paper sack of some coffee grounds and food trash, and then piled the old *Dallas Times Herald* newspapers over the top of that. She would never see them if she took the trash out, but I did that anyway.

I started to cry a little bit when I put the lid on. I couldn't stop myself from it—the tears bouncing off the lid of the galvanized trash can sounded like tiny cymbals of pain. But I had learned how to shut that stuff off pretty quickly by now, so I just choked it down—but I gagged on it a bit.

The seeds of anxiety, depression, and loneliness, liberally sown by all three of us on the fertile ground of a diseased body. It was the perfect setup for anyone to learn how not to handle living with a lifelong disease.

# Alone

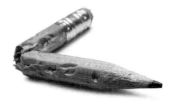

I was learning it was better to be alone. It wasn't how I wanted to be deep inside I felt, and certainly I didn't want to be a loner, but it was much easier. No time around my folks, a little time with a few friends, and most of the time alone.

I wouldn't mess up, act overeager, feel so anxious, or disappoint my parents when I was alone.

It made hiding the sweating and occasional skin problems much easier too.

Things had started to go even worse at home after my second year at elementary school, despite the fact that I had maintained my perfect grades. I was always proud of my academics; neither of my parents seemed to be, at least outwardly when I was around. A friend's mom once complimented me on my continuous series of good grades, which were posted in the hallways and classrooms of our school, during a trip to the grocery store. My mom proceeded to expound on her parental philosophy toward my grade accomplishments with, "We don't expect good grades from W.C.; we demand them!"

I had excelled in both Pop Warner and later official school league football. Football had become my new sport, as I would never play organized baseball again. Football was a much longer season too, with an extra spring practice season to get me out of the house even more.

Then, my guardian angel and protector, my sister, Marcia, decided to get married, removing the referee from our now-routine daily household wars. She just couldn't spend any more of her life in that home and that situation. I understood completely. And I told her I was at the point then where I didn't need any more "protection" either.

"Please go. Have a life. You deserve better," I cried to her in her arms as she left the church after the wedding. She told me, "I'll always be there for you. I swear it," and she always tried to.

Dad gave her a big wedding in 1968, even after spending a great deal of time trying to talk her out of it and finally offering her a six-week trip through Europe with my mom to wait and make sure she still felt the same way when she came back. But I doubt that was much incentive. It seemed to me like six straight weeks with my mom in foreign countries was like last prize in the drawing pool, but my dad was honestly trying to show love and care with that offer, and we all knew it as genuine. Marcia politely and graciously said no. She was getting married, and that was that. He couldn't talk her out of it.

So Colonial Baptist Church, where we belonged and attended regularly (that is to say, Marcia and I attended twice a week, but almost never my mom and never my dad), had a blow-out event of a wedding by any standard. Then, in an instant it seemed, she was gone. Her husband being assigned to military bases around the world meant my guardian angel had moved on. Now, at the age of eleven, I was truly alone, and I was going to have to protect myself.

I had noticed by now I was beginning to develop a temper of my own that was occasionally very difficult for me to control, or even understand, at times. I had heard myself called a bully by a kid from my same class, who was at least as big as me, and it totally took me by surprise. Me, a bully? I honestly had never thought of myself as a bully or rough on other guys, ever.

My symptoms were growing in frequency and severity. The sweating was sometimes out of hand now, requiring me to take a second shirt to school almost every day, rolled up under the seat of my bike. Kids had begun to call my mom "the nut," but only behind my back, never around me or to my face. But I heard about it from H.L., who got into a fight about it with the kid that said it. My mom's moodiness had hit new levels, and she had begun a very maddening and quite hurtful method of surprise slapping me pretty hard but open-handed on the face, back of the neck, or head whenever she lost it for a second. She had also had another "heart attack" incident requiring an ambulance. They were having a real devil of a time diagnosing what was wrong with her. Little wonder, our family disease had not been discovered yet.

Ultimately, they just kept up the trend of raising dosages of more and stronger nervous drugs, like new tranquilizers and sleeping pills, now mixed with some other drugs.

The ferocity of her verbal attacks on me was also noticeably rising in intensity. I was getting just big and mad enough at age eleven now to be about to attack back against either one of my parents, and I think they both knew it. It simply was the best solution to have all three of us apart at that time. We didn't know each other or have any love together anyway.

It would simply be better for everyone if we were all alone.

So Dad and I were on our way now down to San Marcos, Texas, to the military academy I would be attending, beginning in August 1969, as the solution. I hadn't been able to sleep for two days because I was so excited about going. I would finally be away from these people called my parents for weeks, sometimes months, at a time. It was all I could ever hope for.

They told the few friends and family that cared enough to listen that they were sending me there "because the divorce was going to be finalized and it's best if he's away." But I could have cared less about that and had told them so. "What, you think it's some kind of surprise to me you're going to get divorced when you haven't lived together in six years?" I did also tell them occasionally, especially when I was angry or really wanted to make a point that hurt, that I just wanted to be away from *them*. I realize now that they tried to do just that for me, in the best way they could in 1969.

The academy was really a great place for me and gave me so many things I needed in my life and needed at just that time. Things like courage, honor, truth, trust, teamwork, self-discipline, and self-reliance. They had great proctors (male floor supervisors from the local college to supervise each dorm room floor), but mostly, they had great active and retired military leaders. These men, many of whom were combat veterans of WW II, Korea, and lately Vietnam, did not only provide the tough love kids like me especially needed at this age but real morals they could pass on in candid, truly incredible life stories. To be honest, up until my time at the academy, I had learned most of my values from watching *The Andy Griffith Show* and hanging around Coach K.

The academy had a nine-hole golf course—where I picked up the game I love to this day—combination indoor/outdoor swimming pool, several tennis courts, its own church and chapel, separate practice and playing fields for football so the playing field always stayed perfect, and a huge gym with at one end what would become my home away from home with an enormous weight room inside.

Many of the other kids (it was both boys and girls at the academy, but only the boys were involved in the military school part) were in a similar boat as I was at home. Kids from broken homes, from parents working overseas on business or oil and gas assignments, and just kids who wanted, or were wanted, to get away from home. You may be surprised to hear that in the three years I attended there, there was only a single incident of any noticeable homesickness from any kid, boy or girl, that I ever heard about. I wasn't the only one who wanted to get away, I knew for sure. It gave me some confidence.

Make no mistake about it, at twelve years old it was pretty tough at first. I was really alone now, a life more like an eighteen-year-old drafted into military boot camp. I had no experience in many of the things everyone was expected to know how to do because I'd had so little in the way of parenting, but it was tough on every other kid at first as well I'm sure.

Cadets, as we were known, had to maintain their own rooms for military officer inspection daily, as well as clean and maintain their rifle and/or saber (if you were good enough to become an officer). Uniforms, brass, and shoes had to be shined and were inspected every single day but Sunday. Make it to meals on time or miss them. Keep your locker perfect with everything folded military style. No candy or snacks of any kind in your room or locker unless in a box from a parent.

Screw up on one or more of these rules, and the cadet was given "tours" by the officers and master sergeants for the following Saturday (unless it was football season; then they did them on Sunday afternoon). "Tours" were one-hour long marches, in fatigues and combat boots, rifle and backpack, up and down the monstrous hill at the back of the campus. I can relate how steep that hill is in one story. Due to road construction around the main entrance to the school one day, we were diverted into the campus the back way. The school's bus could not climb that hill that day until more than half of the students got out. In my three years there, I got one tour, and I never got another, I can tell you.

I met my new mentor in "Coach Mo" the first day I arrived on campus. It was right after my mom helped me unpack in the tiny dorm room that would be home for that year. He was called Coach Mo because he was one-half pure Blackfoot and kept his hair cut in an absolutely perfect mohawk. He was six feet, six inches, but looked much taller. He had played pro ball somewhere in Canada, where he was from, and had maybe one percent body fat on his two-hundred-and-twenty-five-plus pounds.

Coach Mo was a man in charge wherever he was, not just because he was athletic director, head football coach, and absolutely a huge, striking man. He was also the type of man who was in charge even when around retired military officers, green berets, and special forces soldiers. Nobody argued with Coach Mo. It was shut up and listen when he spoke, which was not that much generally unless it was on a football field. Then he would never shut up. And nobody, I mean *nobody*, could ride you during practice like Coach Mo could.

Yet for all of that blustering verbal bashing he could dish out, most around him felt he was a softie inside, that he only screamed and pushed some of the kids to drive their improvement and growth. And he only drove those he cared about and loved. Pro football players on the borderline of making the cut on pro football teams relate the same type of stories. They'll tell you it's a sure sign of "training camp death" when their coaches stop screaming at them during practice. They know they haven't suddenly gotten it perfect to their coach's quiet satisfaction; rather, they've been given up on.

I knew that feeling. I believed it much better to be ridden like a rented mule.

Only a few days after I arrived at the academy, another incident happened.

Football players have to arrive on campus earlier than the other cadets due to spring training. On the fourth day of spring training, I hadn't been feeling well all day. I was very nervous for no reason and had some nausea and way too much energy. I felt itchy too. I took my turn with the middle school kids in the morning weight room session then broke for lunch. I felt better during the exercise session, but I could hardly eat anything at lunch.

Middle school didn't have an afternoon football practice that day, so it was a free afternoon just a few days before the start of school. Most of the middle school team went to a movie in town. Some high school kids were in the weight room after lunch just messing around. I was full of so much energy, I grabbed the lat machine and began to do reps, and then I moved to bench press, then curls, all around the entire route of the weight machine, every single station, fanatically working myself to the point of exhaustion.

As I stood up from the rowing station, the final station of the weight machine system, I just completely lost my breakfast and lunch, all at once and without warning. It flew *everywhere* in the weight room: the lockers, floor, walls, even on the weight machine itself. When I could finally stand up straight after the dry heaves, dizzy and lightheaded as could be, I saw Coach Mo just staring at me, standing next to the high school kids. I never even knew he had come in. The weight room was Coach Mo's baby; he had personally raised the money for the equipment from two parents just the previous spring.

Oh no, I had lost it ... again.

And I thought, *Oh my God, he's gonna kill me!*

He walked straight over to me from across the room, grabbed me by my shirt just below the neck from behind, and actually picked me up off my feet by accident, my feet dangling like a cartoon character. Then he screamed over at his high school athletes, "If you punks worked out like this kid does, we'd never lose a game!" He let me back down to my feet (he didn't really mean to raise me up; he was just that incredibly strong—and excited too). He slapped me hard on the butt with a really loud pop and, with a look of real respect, shouted just as loud as he could right in my face, "By God, that's the way to work out, man!"

Coach Mo turned to the high school kids, still watching, and he hollered at them, "Get the janitor; you aren't doing anything anyway." They gave me a look that would melt a glacier, but all of them started out of the weight room to get a janitor to clean up the mess. Coach Mo asked me to come up to his office on the third floor of the massive gym complex. Coach Mo was the varsity football coach and athletic director. There were three levels of coaches between Coach Mo and myself, but he wanted to chat a second.

I realize now that that time he spent with me was to make sure I was okay and not going to have a seizure or something. I think he may have been around pro athletes in hockey and football that had similar problems, and he just wanted to watch me for a few minutes. At the time, I only knew that being the only middle school kid to ever have visited Coach Mo's private office made me incredibly lucky. He wasted time talking about all kinds of stupid stuff, ending up with where and what ball I played in Dallas. When we finished, he told me he enjoyed the time a lot and looked forward to me making use of the weight machine he had worked so hard to get for all the kids. I told him raising that money was awesome, and I would be there a lot.

As we went downstairs, the locker room had been thoroughly cleaned; he checked all around to make sure, and then we headed out the front door of the gym. He told me, "All right, knucklehead, I've got my eye on you; don't screw up—even once!"

The Lord had sent me another guardian angel.

But there's a lot of anxiety for anyone off on their own in a boarding school. Natural anxiety from peer pressure and competition. A much higher academic standard to meet. Many other highly intelligent students around, as well as elite athletes. The raised bar is enough for anybody at twelve years old to have some anxiousness.

But to a diseased hyperthyroid sufferer, routine anxiety is much more intense, and the more the disease grows, the more the intensity of the anxiety grows.

The undiagnosed and unknown thyroid disease had caused the symptoms of nausea, dizziness, and muscle pain to grow nearly in tandem with my body. I would not be able to fight them off completely ever again. They were starting to visibly show, and I was unable to control when the symptoms would erupt like never before.

More reason than ever to be alone.

• •

The next two and a half years were the best of my life up until that time. Great leadership from the military trainers and coaches, especially Coach Mo. No contact, except written, with either parent, and then only Mom with a few letters. In the summers when I went home, my dad had odd jobs for me and I went to football camps, so I rarely saw either of them during my entire three years at the academy.

I had made standard-bearer as a seventh grader and newbie (first-year kid), which was a special honor, notable because I was an underclassman to the many still unranked eighth graders. The standard-bearer is the term for the person who carries their company flag in front of the entire company. There were only two, as middle school only had two companies, and generally the standard-bearers were the bigger and stronger of the eighth grade boys who had not made a rank yet, as well as the fact that the flag was more than twelve feet long and somewhat heavy. No problem for me, though by now I was living in the weight room, and the skinny kid that showed up at the academy in August 1969 was beginning to muscle up.

I made captain my second year, one of the two captains allowed in middle school. It was an achievement to be proud of to this day. There was only one way to make captain at the academy—earn it. It didn't matter who the student knew or was or who their parents were, the retired military officers who ran the academy put the cadet up for promotion based on merit, and it took final approval from an active military officer who personally inspected the candidate privately and individually prior to a command letter being issued. The letter offering cadets a commission at the academy came on real U.S. Army paper and was signed by an active U.S. Army General. It's easy to understand this was a pretty big deal to thirteen-year-old kids.

As a complete surprise to me, both my parents attended the parade/festival that involved the commissioning for the following year. It was one of only two times in my life both of my parents ever attended any event of any kind for me together. I don't know how they found out. I guess the academy sent them a letter or something. I deliberately never told them. So I was totally shocked to see them in the VIP box at the football field/parade grounds. When commissioning began and all new officers (myself included) came forward to receive their officer rank, saber, and roses, I saw them seated in the second row of this special section for parents of kids commissioned that day.

*My gosh, how did they find out, and why come down now?* I fumed. For sure, Mom would blow it on such an important day. *Oh my God, no,* was all I could think about as I was handed my saber from our commandant. I almost dropped it.

They only stayed through lunch and then headed back to Dallas. Mom seemed much better. Turns out, I found out later she had been prescribed a new drug, Valium, and her mood swings were supposedly much better, according to my sister and dad. She acted like a perfect mom at the ceremonies. If they could have ever acted that way together, things would be a whole lot different, I'm telling you. Maybe this was the medicine that could save her!

When I waved good-bye to my folks heading off, I turned around to see Coach Mo in a suit and tie. I had never seen Coach Mo in anything but gray coaches' shorts/pants and our green-colored school shirts. He looked great, and if it's possible, even bigger than he usually looked. He smiled wide with those perfect teeth of his when I saw him. I had my new saber positively gleaming in the afternoon sun and three round, solid, silver circles glowing on my collar now. The symbol of a captain.

He laughed really loud, grabbed me with both hands, squeezed me hard on the shoulders, and said, "All right, knucklehead, don't get on a high horse around here, or I'll squash you. Got it!" I just smiled and almost cried right then, but instead I just said, "Yes, sir!"

I t was a perfect year of life for me. We had two great middle school companies that together won the coveted "Star of Honor" at our inspection that year. That meant that all the kids in middle school could wear a special blue star on the right side of the uniform over their name plate the next year, regardless of whether they were moving up to high school or had another year in middle school. That star was known and more than respected in every military base and academy in the world at that time. I excelled in marksmanship in eighth grade—our first year allowed to use live ammunition—and won three ribbons in that single year in competitions. Turns out that even today, I can shoot quite accurately with rifle, shotgun, or pistol with either hand. Just a lucky blessing.

I made standard-bearer again the following year as a fresh-man. To make standard-bearer that young usually meant a cou-ple of important things to a cadet in military school. It required respect from the officers and master sergeant of your company and the corps, and usually the ruling active military staff had slated you for that same *corps*—the short term used for *corps of cadet commanders*—that literally ran the school their junior and senior years. It involved numerous privileges, especially for a freshman non-com in a world of senior officers.

Some of the privileges of making a standard-bearer were staying in the officer-only dorm with limited supervisors and proctors. In this dorm there were much fewer and more lim-ited inspections, not to mention a completely different policy on food and stuff in your rooms; in fact, cadets could order up meals from the Saber, the local school supply and hamburger joint on campus, and have them delivered after study hall! It was much more private and enjoyable with only one roommate (another standard-bearer) instead of four. The showers/toilets were for four-people setup and much nicer, instead of the stan-dard twenty at a time. Standard-bearers ate at the officers' tables and had private and select drill away from all other cadets with currently active military officers. This was the best that life could be that I could imagine.

Until I took a kid named Baker home with me.

His folks lived just walking distance from my dad's new high-rise luxury apartment in north Dallas, but they would not be home from some exotic vacation until the day after we left for break. Baker asked me if he could come home with me the first night that Easter break, but I told him no, he couldn't. I didn't want this because I always had to stay the first night, following day, and night with my mom, and I could not risk a loudmouth like Baker meeting my mom. I gave him some excuse even after he kept after me. Baker had few friends at the academy, and at the time, most of us would have used the term *smart ass* to describe this totally spoiled-rotten kid.

But I guess he got his parents to call my dad and work it out. In any case, I got notice from my mom he was coming home with me for the first day of Easter break. The next day my dad was coming to pick us up and keep us for one night until Baker's parents' got home.

Of course, Mom blew up like a bomb after about an hour around this kid; frankly, I was ready to as well. His know-it-all, totally spoiled, nothing's good or cool enough attitude blew us both up like a roman candle, but I'd known what this kid was like. My mom didn't, and when she would hit the roof on somebody, especially if it was deserving, it was a real Hiroshima event. I know Baker thought she was insane after that. I hoped not but wondered a bit myself. Her anger and disease had hit a new level while I was away at the academy that year.

My standard-bearer status allowed me to return two days later than most of the cadets from holiday breaks, and when I returned from Easter break, the story of a "nut" crazy mom was all over campus.

I was finished there in my opinion. Even my roommate was avoiding me a bit. I never had a word said about it to my face and never discussed it with anybody, but I was still ruined there I believed. My anxiety level, already elevated every day due to disease, would go ballistic when people were talking about me behind my back in an obvious manner. All I could think to do was to get alone and away from them all. For any other kid, it was probably the type of thing that would blow away in a few weeks. But for a diseased, confused, afraid, and anxious four-teen-year-old, it was something else much more dramatic.

Like Hiroshima? Better for all if I moved along alone. I knew I would be leaving the academy at the end of the year.

• •

My commission letter arrived a few days later. It was an invitation to accept the position as master ser-geant for the corps. That was it then. I was slated for corps com-mand, possibly colonel. No guesswork needed.

I resigned the letter the following morning with the new general that had taken over as commandant of the academy just a few days earlier. He became absolutely enraged.

I told him, "My folks just don't have the money for me to come anymore, General." First he demanded to speak to my father directly, telling me, "We have scholarships for corps-slated officers, young man!" Then he called the dean for a long time, making me wait out in the hall while they talked. Fortu-nately for me, they could not reach my mom or dad that day to confirm the story either. Things were different when he called me back in, and he spoke to me very frankly and directly about overcoming challenges and things like that. I just kept lying like crazy. I was learning how to be a fantastic liar now, as well as a con artist at times. What terrific life skills I was building!

I went straight to Coach Mo at the gym after my visit with the general. I told him I had resigned my letter and would not be returning, my folks just couldn't afford it now, and I was fine with public school. He just looked at me with the kind of look a war hero would give to somebody that had just betrayed their country. I knew right then he knew I was a total liar, and I was totally destroyed inside. The truth was I *was* just running away.

He said, "Okay, knucklehead, just keep running in the right direction," and shook my hand, man to man.

I have never lived down lying to Coach Mo. I never will. It haunts me to this day, as he did not live long enough for me to apologize to.

What I didn't know then, that the dean knew and probably told the general on the phone earlier, was that if my folks could no longer afford my tuition there, then things had greatly changed in their financial situation. Unknown to me or my mom, my dad had donated $15,000 cash for new lights for our football field/parade ground so we could be the only academy in Texas to play night games or have regular night parades. He did it just after my officer commissioning. When I think of the events later, I did remember seeing Coach Mo, my dad, and the dean all together during lunch speaking very privately. At the time, I can just remember hoping my dad would act charming like he did when business was on the line, rather than the way he acted around me and Mom most of the time. Looks like I blew that one. They had already begun installing the lights while I was writing my resignation.

Anyway, it was back to public school—a huge one, with 1,500 kids. Surely I could hide there for three years. Just three more years, and it would be much easier to be happy.

I was sure alone would make it better for all around.

And I had decided now I was through with running away from anything or anybody.

Never again. That would stop this nervousness.

I didn't ask my folks about my decision. I told them I would not be going back for any future years at the academy and had decided to return to public school to graduate with my grade school friends. I had made my contribution to their future happiness by leaving so they could fight out the legal portion of the divorce in private. That was over. They never questioned my judgment. There was no discussion or attempts to persuade me, by any method, to stay at the academy. It wouldn't have worked anyway; I was as tough as they were by then. The family unit had become just like a championship boxing match by now, the three of us circling each other like professional boxers looking for an opening for a right cross. The strongest, most angry, or most drugged at the time would wind up winning the inevitable day-to-day battles that occurred. None of us facing up to the reality that we had all already lost the war.

# The Genesis of Self-Abuse:

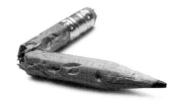

## *Disease, Anxiety, and Depression*

I hid out in high school like Mata Hari. Alone in a sea of 1,500 high school kids.

I spent the first two years with no associations of any kind except those restarted from friendships from elementary school, especially H.L. Bill's family had sent him to Christian Schools Inc., so there were just two of the old gang left at the giant high school by the time I returned. That was perfect, no bad or mouthy kids to have to beat into quiet submission (yes, I guess I was turning into a bully, and officer training in military school had only reinforced that). But I allowed nobody else but H.L. or Bill near either parent, especially my mom. Things went very well for almost the full three years.

The Valium drug was working pretty well on Mom's moodiness and attitude. My mom had also gotten a job as a home-mortgage loan closer at a large firm downtown. That required some pretty late hours sometimes, and with my sports and my own new job at the car wash, we hardly saw each other.

I killed them at the car wash with my adrenal energy that

never stopped, good manners, and years of experience cleaning the family car. I honestly can tell you I got a raise on my second day of employment there. I also made more tips than anybody in the facility. Most guys wanted to work the wipe-down area, or where the car first comes out of the automated machine wash. It's pretty simple and easy work to give the car its first wipe down and then drive it to the gas pumps/vacuum station. But there was no tip money in that job.

I learned where and how the tip money was made pretty fast. I was constantly sweating, even in the wintertime, and could clean the inside of a car really well—pretty quickly too. I would jump in and out of the car, looking like I had just put 110 percent into it, give a very polite line of bull as the customer paid, hold the car door open, and *wham*—the money just came flying out of their pockets for me. After my second week there, I was making double my hourly salary in tips alone. H.L. told me more than a year after I quit there—having quit only at my mom's multiple tearful requests to try to work it out with my dad—that people were still driving up and asking for that "Clay kid" to do their car. I had surely learned how to use my diseases for money. Having a good sweat that was almost always up, even when between cars or in the winter, plenty of energy, and a drive for perfection can help you earn an extra buck or two at anything, especially something like a car wash or service business. Who cares exactly what the root cause is; cash is way more important when you're fifteen and want to buy your first car.

I also found out right after my sophomore year and the first of three straight years I would earn National Honor Society for maintaining a 4.0 average (public high school was just a joke compared to the academic program at the academy) that many of the kids, especially some of the girls, if you can believe it, were talking about me as "conceited," "aloof," and "unapproachable." My God, if they only knew.

Of course, I did or said nothing to divert those views. It was a perfect cover.

Because I had already learned it was easiest to be alone.

You see, my own problems with my adrenaline, anxiety, and thyroid disease were beginning to grow rather strongly again, just like my body was. I was starting to have concerns that persisted for many years that both my mom and I had mental illness. We were both far too angry, far too demanding, and far too anxious for everything to be all right with us. At the time, the only place one could go to discuss this type of behavior was a psychiatrist. I knew I didn't want to see a psychiatrist, and for sure my mother wouldn't. There was not only a real social stigma attached to that in the early 1970s, but it might mean facing a terribly ugly truth as well.

The issues and consequences of denial and fear many times go hand in hand.

One of the problems that developed with this combination of symptoms caused by thyroid disease, at least with me, was a lack of confidence that must be hidden from view. This lack of personal confidence, despite any successes already achieved, can cause a sufferer to be unable to take any rejection, and if given any, it will be taken as personal, a direct affront to their belief system. Anxiety, especially when combined with a lack of confidence like I was experiencing, wouldn't allow someone with my combination of conditions to accept any argument or alternative point of view from anybody except a superior officer (there were no superior officers in public school, and frankly, after three years of private-school-quality teachers, I thought most of our teachers were lucky to hold their jobs). As a previous officer and standard-bearer, I had learned in those years of military school leadership not to even tolerate a different point of view. It was my way or the highway—period. There wasn't another option.

Sooner or later, no matter how smart, handsome, intimidating, or athletic you are, somebody's going to test that sorry attitude out. I had mine tested by a varsity lineman a couple of inches taller and about forty pounds or so heavier than me at the end of my sophomore year at a school general assembly. I had come out before him, turned to wait on a couple of buddies, and he started it.

It was a simple push to my chest, even backhanded as if to swat away a fly, to move me out of a senior's way—not a deliberate shove, just an attitude movement, kind of showing off for his girlfriend. I had experienced and had had to take that stuff before at the academy. You might have to take it there because if that boy was an officer, you could be kicked out of school for striking him, starting a fight, and other very strict rules. But not here in public school. I knew that.

So I turned away and began to apologize for being in his way and then immediately turned back. I got both my arms under his armpits in a split second and began to drive him right back into the assembly hall with my head under his chin (this was hand-to-hand combat training 101 at the academy), knocking boys, girls, and teachers flying behind us along the way down the assembly aisle as I was driving him backward maybe ten or more rows into the hall. Despite his size and weight advantage, he was completely unable to stop what was happening to him. I drove him straight and hard in a perfect-form tackle over the back of those assembly chairs that have the swing-up seats in them (you remember the old wood ones that made your butt sore after about thirty minutes). The force of my head under his chin drove the back of his head against the seat of that wooden chair and knocked him out cold. Then I began, quite calmly I can remember, to slam the wooden seat back and forth against his head just as hard as I could in an attempt to crush his skull.

I had completely lost it again. It took about five or six kids, plus two teachers, to drag me off him, H.L. told me later. H.L. didn't try to help stop it though.

Fortunately, several kids had seen me be pushed first and told the powers that be how it all got started. I never even got called to the principal's office over it. I guess that's partially because I had never been in any trouble before then and partially because they had to call an ambulance for the senior first. I never saw him again. I don't know if he was able to graduate; the ceremonies were only a few weeks away.

I had now had two major fights in my life, had lost it both times, and had sent both, by ambulance, to a hospital. I thought to myself, even then at fifteen years old, that this was a really bad trend. But I quickly rationalized those thoughts away. *I never started either of these fights. It's not my fault,* I could tell myself, and that made it much easier to choke down and quickly forget the fear that I could be a bit "off" myself.

Many of the kids who saw what happened just couldn't forget and didn't, but because the senior I fought with was known as a real jerk anyway, the incident slowly just went away. But I noticed some looks at me in the halls had definitely changed. As a result of those looks, I began to walk straight down the middle of that giant high school's halls between classes like a direct challenge, with every single person, male or female, getting out of my way from the next day until the day I graduated. "Don't even think about messing with me" was the message.

I guess they got it. Nobody ever decided to test my attitude again.

It also helped make sure one had a lot of time alone.

The reality is my medical problems were making me act as a conceited, know-it-all, menacing bully, despite how I wanted to act and be thought of. And I kept thinking, *This just isn't me! I'm not this way!* But the honest truth was that it was much, much easier to be thought of and act that way than to be thought of and act like the son of a crazy mom, a crazy kid, or show just how scared, nervous, and—now I know but didn't know then—just how sick I really was.

The fear of having a girl meet my parents combined with my anxiety over rejection meant I never had a single date until my senior year. I guess that was because I refused to ask even one girl out. To much chance at the whole dating thing revealing both my own as well as my family's problems, I thought. Besides, I hadn't met anyone worth all the risks.

Just as my sophomore year began, I began restoring a cherry red, 1968 convertible SS Camaro I had just bought with every dime I had made and saved in my year and a half at the car wash. It had been wrecked when I bought it, but the engine and transmission were sound, so I got a really good deal. I told myself that I had no money right then for dates, even though I had to be making a fortune for a fifteen-year-old kid at the car wash. I had already ordered the giant Mickey Thomson fifty-inch rear tires and four custom chrome wheels for that car that cost over three hundred bucks alone in 1974. This baby had a four speed on the floor, the famous .327 Chevy small block, a four barrel Holley "big throat" carb, and was a convertible too. By my junior year, it was one of, if not *the* most, envied car in the more than one-thousand-car parking lot of our high school.

I would be getting my license right before the start of my junior term and would have one hell of a ride to cruise to school in next year! Let's see what everyone thought and how they looked at me then.

I was completely devastated beginning my first day of classes my senior year. A third torn ACL in my left knee had ended my football career permanently six days before school began in spring training, as well as any chances at any college scholarship—even junior colleges. They wanted to do surgery immediately, but I nixed that and nixed it good. Why bother? Let me just go to school and finish my senior year as best I can without falling behind from the get-go being out of school for several weeks after the surgery. "I'll get it done after graduation," I said. I still haven't.

But all that despondency ended right away when I saw the angel sitting up two rows and on my left in third period honors English class that first day.

I had never seen her before in school, but she had been there—in different classes than me—for two years. She joked with me later that she had gone from what she called an "ugly duckling" to what I called about the hottest thing in life over the last summer.

I went from a guy who hadn't even considered a date to wanting one more than a football scholarship in about thirty seconds.

I stole a look at the class roll right before class and found out her name was Wendy. She was about five feet eight inches tall, weighed about 125, and had a gorgeous figure with very full and thick long light-brown hair almost to her waist. She also had the most beautiful set of legs I had ever seen on any woman alive. Even movie stars. It also seemed that that whole first day in class, by accident or not, she seemed to aim and tilt them just where I could stare at them in perfect view. Friends, I couldn't tell you one word said that day in class; all I could do was gaze at those incredible legs the entire fifty-five minutes. I was so disappointed to hear the bell ring I swear I almost moaned out loud.

When class was over, she seemed to need a half second to gather her things and rise, so I hobbled up on the good knee as quickly as I could and tried as casually as possible when I limped by to say, "Hey, Wendy. See you tomorrow?"

She said, "Wait a second, Clay." (I had begun to use my middle name, Clay, when I came back from military school instead of the initials W.C. that I had grown up with and my dad went by too.)

Oh yeah? Maybe an opening! And I didn't think she even knew I was alive.

Turns out, she had seen me around some.

She wanted to know what my schedule was, and we shared those, none of which matched because I tutored two classes to complete a commitment that would get me into a very rare internship for high school students in the second semester. She tutored other classes, including honors math. We did have the same lunch period—the early lunch always for seniors—and we agreed to meet then for lunch. We talked long enough to be late for third period. I can't remember about what.

We were together constantly from that point on.

The only mistake Wendy, or her incredibly beautiful family for that matter, ever made was loving and trusting in me. In return for their love, trust, and caring, I repaid them by misleading, deceiving, and lying to them at every single important time to cover up what was becoming a very serious problem with my mom and a growing problem with me: our thyroid diseases and our resulting behavior and anxiety problems.

And, of course, my ego, which had now grown to a size just slightly smaller than Canada.

Unknown to either my mom or me, my sister was having some pretty tough times herself.

But the next two and a half years were really a fantastic and loving time … mostly.

● ●

The internship I earned through the National Honor Society grading and selection process was a fantastic and really fun way for students to learn things they could never learn in any school, anywhere. If one of your kids or friends' kids ever gets a chance at this, please encourage them to do it; it's more than worth it.

Most of the high school internships today are very developed and structured programs that allow students to work side by side, day to day during regular work hours instead of attending class at high school, usually at the senior grade level. Our program began with executive internships because it was executives initially that donated funds to establish the program with the Dallas Independent School District. Students would spend Monday through Thursday usually right in the office of, or right next to the office of, a business executive in the Dallas area. This is happening in most school districts today in one form or another; it may be that it's not so focused on executive training.

The program I was in was in its infancy, only its second term, and still working out the details, but one really good thing already was in place. The executives sent your grades in, not the teachers. Students in the program would only go to school for their athletics, band, or specific extracurricular programs for an entire semester. The executives in our program became the nine-to-five "teachers" in every sense. It really kept the student in line and coming to work every day, as well as keeping the business executive assessing their impact and growth on a regular basis.

I had developed the "posse," or more usually nicknamed by the other intern mates as "Clay's Girls," for the Friday weekly meetings we held with the internship supervisor for the Dallas Independent School District. We would have a meeting every Friday morning, at unusual places around the city, one time the zoo, the next time the executive floor of the Mobil building downtown. Our school was the only school that had placed three people in the program, which was made up of just twenty-five total students from around the whole city of Dallas in 1975.

The "girls" and I would travel, always together, to each Friday meeting for more than just a show for my ever-increasing ego; they would make sure they had "appointments" or I would have a "meeting" to get to by 3 p.m. That's because I had started a full-time job with an oil-drilling equipment maker to help me pay for part-time college, and I had to get to work (neither the internship program nor the school system knew or would allow this). But they weren't just the girls or anything as simple as that to me. They were Deborah and Patty, two more guardian angels of my life. I love them both to this day, but there was never any dating; we all had separate boy and girlfriends. That made it a very special relationship for us all.

That fact was not lost on the other interns or on the intern coordinator.

Halfway into the initial year of the program, Deborah and I were selected for an interview with the *Dallas Morning News* newspaper about our internship. It turned into a large feature with pictures for the Sunday front page of the *Dallas Morning News* business section. Handling the media with a big bunch of "give 'em a grin and a positive spin" seemed very simple and came completely naturally.

The program tripled in size the next semester. In two years, it had over a thousand interns. Internships with businesses have become an enormous success all across the country.

The new job at the oil-drilling equipment manufacturer was also the reason that I picked the particular company I selected for my internship. Frankly, not because I thought I would necessarily learn something that would help me down the line by working with them, even though I did some I'm sure; but it was because their intern supervisor would also let me go around three or so, and I could make it to my new full-time job.

There were a great bunch of executives at this firm I was interning at, but my dad and his business operations were so far ahead of this giant company it was a joke. I mean, these guys had a meeting about meetings about the meeting they were going to have to plan the annual meeting. But it was really cool in all honesty; they flew me to corporate events on their private jet, had the most outrageous parties I ever saw in my life, and in general, gave me a very thorough taste of the corporate good life.

It was a taste I will never forget.

Things were about to change though. I hadn't blown it with Wendy yet, but the final escape from my mom was just around the corner.

• •

It was just over a couple of weeks before graduation, a Saturday in May I think. My mom's moodiness had come back lately—at times worse than ever before—and even stronger dosages of Valium and some other new drugs were not helping her. She had begun to age very badly. Far beyond her forty-five years of age in appearance, she was beginning to look over sixty, and remember, this was a very beautiful model at one time.

Her hair was terrible, her nails were constantly breaking, and the skin problems had come back for her as well.

The numbers of misdiagnoses she got were just over the top. First the false heart attacks, then the bowel troubles; then they addressed the nerves for the rest of her life, never trying to slow the ever rising amount of dosage with stronger medications. They simply had no clue. One time diabetes was sure to be it, but no. Then another time, just like me later in life, it was arthritis, but no. Then it was something else, on, and on, and on. Always wrong.

I just honestly didn't know that or what was really going on in the summer of 1975. But I would have given anything to— especially now.

Mom had begun to gain weight now, and that was making her freak out. She had always prided herself on her model-like figure, and for some reason, she had lost all control of her weight. She had gone to skipping all meals during the day and then only eating very lightly in the early evening.

This is also exactly what I have begun to do myself; the only difference is I understand why and do it after the benefit of medical consultation. With some folks who suffer thyroid and metabolic disorders, proper digestion of food will only take place at certain times of the day. Eating during the "wrong" time or eating the "wrong foods" means the body will get very little nutritional benefit from the calories taken in. They will just be stored as fat. I needed help from a doctor, dietitian, *and* a nutritionist to figure out both when and what I can eat.

I believe Mom was instinctively trying to match her food intake to her metabolism times like I've learned to just take a light amount of fruit during the day when I'm hungry. I know I can usually eat and metabolize a full meal after about 3 p.m. But like all advanced thyroid disease sufferers, I've got to listen to my body first. It will tell me when I can eat and when I shouldn't. Not only is every sufferer's metabolic disorder different, sufferers will learn that for certain periods during their life, they're different day to day.

Mom joined a gym in a very nice part of town but always needed a ride there, as Mom had never driven a car in my lifetime. She had said it was "doctor's orders" due to her heart. But I know now it was simple anxiety pumping up the thyroid, causing her to fear driving. I didn't know that back then, but I didn't mind taking or picking her up anytime she needed it. She had to work with me on this though. Saturday was a good work day for me, all overtime. So I need to finish my full shift at 3 p.m., and then I would pick her up.

"You better be there when I finish at 3:30!" she screamed at me.

I told her, "Catch your own ride to an' fro; see ya," and headed for the door. She settled down, asked for a second to compose herself, then asked politely for a ride and said to just come when I got off work. I said, "Sure; no problem." But I have to say, in retrospect, that after about eleven consecutive years of this, I was getting very short on patience with her, and everybody else too for that matter. Especially right then.

Even with a jet I couldn't have made it from the part of town I worked to the upscale part of Dallas her exercise club was at by 3:30, but I hustled it up and made it about 3:45 or so.

She came out with such a nice smile, I remember, and looked like she'd had a great workout when she came out of the club, waved at some other ladies just leaving, and headed for the

Camaro. I reached over to open the door for her as I was still seated in the driver's seat.

That's when she hit me again—for the last time—screaming, "I told you to pick me up by 3:30!"

Now a lady's gym bag is not a killer weapon, but the shoes hit right across my eyes and nose, and that really made me beyond mad. Had she been anybody else, man or woman, I would have beaten her to death right there in the middle of the parking lot with my bare hands.

But I was just through with her now. Not running away, like Coach Mo had said, but through with her.

I quickly closed the door, pulled a $20 bill out of my wallet, threw it at her out the window, told her to call herself a cab, and drove off. I could see her in my rearview mirror just staring at me in disbelief. As of today, I don't know if the disbelief was from my driving off or from how terribly she had just acted.

And that was the next to last time I ever saw my mother, dead or alive.

Mom's disease had made her an unbearable stress factor to me, without either of us being able to understand why. I knew in my heart it was best we were alone from each other but had trouble expressing the nasty truth of it to anybody, including myself. In reality she desperately needed me, or someone, to help her deal with a disease still undiscovered. I couldn't have done it if my life depended on it though. I couldn't even help myself.

I headed straight home. Graduation was only a few weeks away, and I didn't need to live at her house anymore. I had a friend who had graduated just the previous term and had a cheap two-bedroom apartment only a couple of miles away. I called him and asked him if he'd found any roommates yet. He said no, he hadn't tried that hard, but could use some money, and said, "Hey, what's going on man?"

"I'm moving out. Now. This minute. Can I come there, and I will help pay?"

He said, "Sure; come on."

I packed up my military school duffel with mostly work clothes, underwear, socks, a few decent things to wear around Wendy, and shoes. I also took the approximately $285 I had in cash—all I had—and left.

It wasn't much to start with, but I thought nothing could be worse than where I was.

Later, I would arrange to get all my other things, especially the rifles I had won in competitions, out of the house and into Wendy's garage.

I was really, really worried about my mom, but I just had to choke that down.

I also felt freer than at any time I could remember in my life.

But I felt like something was still wrong with me. I was free but not ... not calm. I had "gotten away" from one big problem in my mom, only to face an even more dangerous issue—depression.

# Becoming a Liar

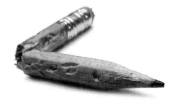

I did not tell Wendy that I had moved out, or anybody else for that matter.

Why bother now? I had been lying or concealing the truth from her virtually since day one of the relationship. Small lies at first, then growing as one gets caught in old cover-ups, or the problem(s) become bigger and impossible to hide. Anxiety may cause the lying or covering up to start, but it turned out that fear and denial would become the backbreaking straws.

I knew it was always easier to be alone, but after Wendy and I came together, suddenly there was a big problem with that—I realized being alone is lonely. But telling her some of the ugly truths might have run her off before we could get started.

So it started with small lies, like covering up why my mom or dad were never available for any of our school functions or time with Wendy's parents (I didn't want them there and never told them or offered an invitation was one reason, just not a reason I shared with Wendy). They grew from there to occasional health cover-ups, like when a skin issue would suddenly pop up. Heaven forbid I would discuss anxiety. I was sure it would appear far too weak in her eyes, and that was an unacceptable option.

I justified the deception and lies to someone I cared about by rationalizing that everybody has a few skeletons in the closet.

The only problem with that thought process is as deception and denial start to grow, eventually the closets will start bursting out and the rooms will fill up. It eventually winds up leaving one nowhere to go.

But being lonely was horrible too. I dreamed our relationship would stay afloat despite the doubts I had about keeping all the plates spinning that I'd started.

The school finals and internship were finished, and seniors were now on half day till the end of the school year, so it was no problem for Wendy and I to do our tutoring in the mornings (by the second semester of senior year, honors students only did teaching or the special internship, as they should have long ago completed any required classes) and then have lunch every day together. It made life worth living; in fact, it was wonderful really.

The senior prom was a dream. I had saved enough for a limousine to take us. Wendy had been nominated for "Most Poised" in the school, which basically meant she was the most desirable young woman in the school in every way. She lost out to a fantastic blonde who was great too—don't get me wrong—but nothing like Wendy. But neither of us cared much at all about it. Wendy was just way too big for that, and, more than just poised, she saw right through me and a lot of my bull from day one and acted like it was nothing more than a fly on the wall. Truly, an unbelievable lady I still haven't given enough credit to.

I had had no contact with my mom for almost two months and more than a year with my dad. All I wanted from them now was to be left alone. There was a chance to work my way up the ladder at the oil field manufacturer that had, unbelievably, given me a full-time job at seventeen. They had given me this opportunity while I was lying straight to their faces about my age and school status. I had originally gotten my job there as temporary/part time, doing what was known as "yard man" work (low on the totem pole but good money) during my internship. But I desperately had to have this full-time job now to pay rent and part-time college expenses. I mean, I just *had* to have it. I didn't care if it was in the "yard" or not.

This company, as a hard policy, would never hire anyone under eighteen or who was still in high school for full-time work. The hiring manager was giving me the eye something serious, but this time, I didn't blink one bit. He gave me one of the breaks of my life. A chance in the sheet metal mechanic shop, one of the most desirable jobs available in that company without a college degree, or in any manufacturing outfit like this one for that matter, in 1976. I guess that man knew desperation and commitment when he saw it.

I wasn't a born liar I hoped, but I knew I was turning into a good one. I had to be; the deceptions were turning into a full-time job by themselves.

Don, the sheet metal shop foreman, especially found out I was a complete liar. I let something slip out during our grueling two-hour final interview. But he signed off on my full-time hiring to come into his most desirable shop and elite shift of mechanics in the whole company, saying the oddest thing to me as I left: "We've been down some of the same trails together, Clay." It took years for me to figure that one out. Finally I did, only it was at his funeral about eight years later after talking at length with his widow.

But for now, the Lord had sent me another guardian angel even though I didn't possibly deserve it.

The lack of stress from my mom had helped me some with my own anxiety and thyroid issues initially when I moved out. But they were returning and, if possible, were getting a little worse. But awesome energy at a new job with highly impressionable people can work in your favor pretty well, especially if you could hide that something was wrong, like the classic 1930s con man I was learning to be.

● ●

A giant manufacturing operation like the one I worked for in the mid-1970s had its own style and manner of "pecking order." Those that worked in the offices were not expected to come to the shops and get dirty or do manual work. Those that worked in manufacturing had their pecking order by grade, or pay grade: yard grade guys at the bottom, machinists and sheet metal grade mechanics at the top.

I was started as painter's helper, grade two. (Yeah, they only had one grade lower in the sheet metal shops.)

But grade two in the sheet metal shop paid out at about grade five anywhere else, and almost double the yard pay, so I couldn't care less. There was not actually any painting done until much later at assembly. The painting we did in our shop was to simply primer the metal to reduce the rust factor, as most of the parts were so large they had to be stored out of doors. When final assembly was readied for the oilrig, the parts were painted with a glossy enamel yellow paint, decals put on, and sent back to assembly and packaging.

The paint area was a total mess on my first day; the three guys on second shift currently in paint department could obviously care less about what they were doing, and it showed. It was filthy, disorganized, and a bunch of the equipment didn't even work (that was a sin at a company like this that always kept *everything* in perfect working order). The worst part of it though was the total lack of job pride, or what I have always called "ownership," in that group of guys. Their workspaces exhibited it better than anything else could. I equated it to them on a personal level, a prejudging personality failure I have always had that almost immediately shows itself to the other party.

They didn't care for me much either for that matter, and right away too.

I had long ago learned to care less about that stuff. I began first, without instruction from them, Don, or anybody else for that matter, to begin to clean up and rebuild the paint guns so we could at least have a full-working equipment group and all guys could actually work at one time! I wondered to myself a little about Don, *Why is he putting up with this?* I learned later that it was the best he could get.

Don never gave me a single instruction, order, or assignment. He just came out at times and watched.

One of the employees tried in kind of a half-hearted attempt to "train" me how to take apart the paint guns when it was obvious what I was going to do. But I had tutored shop for two straight years in high school and had painted a couple thousand hand-built parts by this time, so I just said, "Oh, you mean like this?" as I stripped it down in about six seconds in front of him. I can be quite a conceited jerk at times, but he honestly had it coming.

He just walked off, never said a word or spoke to me again. He quit a couple of weeks later.

It was over an hour and a half before the first primer was sprayed that shift. I thought to myself, *This is nuts!* And the work was backing up like crazy from just our shift alone.

On my second day, after the lines and paint guns were cleaned and operative, I came into shift about twenty minutes early and caught the one paint crewman that was on first shift. They only had one man to paint that shift's parts because they were a smaller group, did much smaller projects, and did not have the daily overtime demands. He thanked me several times for the maintenance work and admitted he didn't really know how to do it, as he'd had no lead man to train him in the three weeks he had been employed. He learned fast though. I showed him in less than fifteen minutes. From that day on until I went to the coast to work a little over a year later, there was never a gun or line down in the paint department—ever.

The paint area was one of the largest of the whole shop, probably because the finished hand-built machinery was always backing up. They had built a series of large hydraulic cranes along one side to move and then store the very large parts, and had a conveyor rail for the small to midsized parts. The trouble was the finished products were all stacked in disorder, and "rush" jobs, with a special tag, weren't getting rushed, as they were stuck in the pile of routine work and not going out to the customer, even though they were completed and just needed priming prior to shipping.

I began to use the central hoist and started pulling out all the rush orders from the mess. I moved about six of these into paint position at the start of the shift, and the lead painter four hollered over at me, "What do you think you're doing?"

I told him I was prepping the rush orders to go out first and that most of these had been there at least the two days I had worked there.

He said, "You're a grade two helper; you just do what I tell you to do, and shut up unless spoken to."

He wasn't that tough. I knew it, and I think he did too, but he thought he could bluff me off. I told him, "Why don't you sneak out back for another sherm (a *sherm* was the street term at that time for a cannabis-laced cigarette) and help us both out because I don't want to lose my job for breaking your stupid neck! Got it?"

That was when Don stepped out from behind a huge chain guard a few feet away. I don't know how long he had been there; nobody else did either. That chain guard was well over eight feet tall, and you could hide a pickup truck behind it.

He asked the painter four, who was the lead painter, to come to his office and bring his cigarettes.

He left Don's office, with timecard in hand, about twenty minutes later.

*Terrific. On the job two days, got one guy canned, another quits in less than two weeks. What leadership and what a fantastic way to make friends on my new job,* I worried. *God, can't I cool it anywhere?*

Actually, it worked the other way, as these types of things sometimes do. The mechanics, doing very dangerous work on huge press brakes, punch machines, and rollers, needed help from the paint crew due to the size of the work involved, even with a crane to help. Nobody wanted a drinker or a doper on the other end of a machine that could get you killed in less than a second. Respect from the real craftsmen in that shop went up about tenfold for me in a single day. Frankly, I was just hoping I wasn't ruined there, as I needed that job and wasn't going to quit.

The painter three that was left didn't talk to me much anymore until after I got my apprentice, but he would work and do as he was told. That was enough. Within a couple of months, we turned out to be pretty good friends.

We cleared up the backlog in about two weeks after I began full-time work. But my sweating problems were becoming noticed by my coworkers and foreman. It was early spring, and it had been unusually cool for that time of the year in Dallas. The paint crew worked directly in front of a sixteen-foot by twenty-five-foot door, open all the time due to the noxious fumes despite a strong ventilation system in the work area itself. Don came out fairly early one shift, before dark, and commented, "You're working yourself into a frenzy, Clay; it's freezing here, and you're sweating." But he did not mean it as a joke, like he had tried to say it, I knew. It was a serious and probing question. But I was way past getting tricked that easily.

I thought I was too fast a liar for Don. I told him I was helping Chris on walls (the "wall" table, which was a very tough welding table and in the warmest part of the building) for the whole start of the shift. He thought for a minute, then nodded, and then just walked away. Problem was, Chris was still doing layout on the walls (a strictly solo-type job where you lay out the job with a colored grease marker all over the steel before you begin to build); the welding was still a couple of days away yet—and Don knew it.

Liars always get caught, eventually, on every lie. I just thought I was a better liar than anybody else. I wasn't, not even close—yet.

I found out later that day where Chris was on his job and resolved then to learn exactly where everybody was at the start of their shift, or I was going to be found out. Don was just too smart to fool for ten to twelve hours a day.

At the end of my ninety-day probationary period, I was promoted to painter four—lead painter for both shifts, two levels being the most you could go until the next review without a special exemption from the office. Don also placed me in the apprentice one line to become the next apprentice when a table opened up to become a mechanic.

●　●

I was losing the battle of lies with Wendy. Or rather, my battle to keep her trust.

We were at that point in the relationship that demanded some commitment, one way or the other. That left me no way out of an impossible corner. Exposing all the lies I had been committing for our entire relationship with some sort of ridiculous mea culpa seemed beyond belief for a real future together. How could she ever forgive me for something like that? I wondered to myself if even I would forgive her for something like that. I couldn't positively say I could do it without doubt. So I just kept trying to hold us together, without exposing the problems that were growing both with me, my mom, and still unknown to any of us, my sister.

I could not lose Wendy now; she was way too important. Any lie, any amount of money, time, whatever, to keep her by me for now was what I would do. I mean *anything*.

The stupidest and most obvious problem with that ridiculous strategy was that she was never given a chance.

But that's what I did, until it eventually blew up, as you knew it would.

∙ ∙

The next incident was kind of anticlimactic really. One early afternoon around 5 p.m., we just ran out of work to paint, rack, and stack, as they say. Two (instead of the union-desired four) guys overcame nineteen guys' ability to build; it was that simple really.

I headed straight for Don's office and knocked on the door. "Why are you holding work from us? Our lines are empty," I demanded, rather curtly too, especially for a painter four to his foreman.

He just gave me a confused look and then said, "We're not holding back anything at all! Let me get Jim (the lead man) and find out what's going on. Hey. What happened to that full line of parts you got late last night?" he asked.

I didn't know what to say; they were just done. But Don was giving me the eye something serious. The painter three had been sick all week. I had been the only one there for two days.

The truth was they weren't going to have that much work finished and ready for paint that day, or probably for another day as well. I was to go to a mechanic's table that I liked and help them with their work order.

Only I was to stay in the office for just a second, privately, with Don.

Uh-oh.

Don just stared at me. Did not say a word. After Jim, the lead man, came in a couple minutes later, he sat down with Don, and they handed me a ridiculously simple set of plans for a chain guard made from .14 gauge steel, average size material. The job was a joke; maybe eight mounting holes clearly laid out for one-half-inch bolts, a cover cut like a bicycle chain cover, and a flange for bolt up. I could have done this job with a piece of roofing tin, a punch, and a ball peen hammer.

Don said, "Can you build that?"

I said, "I think it would be better in .12 gauge, a bit heavier material, but I can build all you want; do you want more than one?"

He gave me a pretty hard but respectful look then said, "Oh, you're an engineer too? Take Randy's table; he's out for his surgery. Let me see what you've got; just one—if it's not too much of a bother, sir."

Okay, okay, point made. I asked him if it was okay if I used the manual brake for the bending. I was a bit scared of the giant hydraulic press brake the real mechanics had slowly begun to use, and I didn't know how to set the angles with the die system that was coming into vogue now. I also didn't want to waste a mechanic's time to help me do a test job. It was much easier with the old equipment, like Mr. Shipp had, especially for me. He just said, "You're the mechanic; don't forget to punch in, but do you need us to shear it for you first, sweetheart?" That was a bit of a taunt in our industry. To "shear" something in a mechanics' shop was to use the giant hydraulic shears to cut the gross materials of eight-feet-by-four-feet steel down to exact size and very tight tolerance. Being a shear man was a starter job, not for mechanics. Mechanics were not expected to waste time cutting down large sheets of steel to later build.

I punched back. "No, I think I can do this with stuff out of your scrap pile; it's plenty big enough." Touché, buddy.

The company had recently gone to IBM-type punch cards you used with your personal ID card to time how long each process of your assigned assembly project was taking: how long for layout, precision cutting, bending and/or rolling, welding, etc. This was what they used to figure everything from how much to charge for something to how much it cost to build, and everything else down that line.

I didn't know it then but found out soon that the punch card timing system was going to be both my best friend and worst enemy. I sure was a paradox coming right at them too.

I went to Randy's table, the shop steward, even though we were an open union shop, and went to work.

A "table" in a precision-sheet-metal shop is sort of like having a corner office at the law firm—in a manufacturing facility way, especially a shop like this. In actuality, you had a perfectly flat, machined, solid-steel table of between ten feet by ten feet to fifteen feet by thirty feet, depending upon your specialty after you finished your apprenticeship and the size of jobs you were assigned.

The lead man assigned your jobs based on a myriad of things like rush, priority, stock, and what he knew the individual skills and likes and dislikes of each mechanic in the shop. It was a very physically demanding and highly individualistic job where the mechanics took extraordinary pride in their finished work product.

You received each job assignment on a routine wood pallet, with raw steel of varying thickness cut to very close tolerance. Along with that was a plastic packet with an IBM punch card and the drawings for what you were to build. Beyond that, you had nothing. You built it your own way to exact tolerances, and then it was inspected. If it failed (and you would receive total hell from your fellow mechanics when you had a return), you corrected it or rebuilt it, counting toward the previous time spent on the job. But believe me, the trouble from your buddies if you got a return was a heck of a lot more painful than any time count the office would add.

At your individual table, you had virtually anything and everything possible to build steel machine parts. You had your own welding machine, torch and burning setup, overhead crane, air pressure lines, hydraulic lines and equipment, at least one giant tool chest, but most had three or four for your own personal tools you were expected to buy as you progressed up the grading ladder. However, the company provided everything else: drill bits, punch dies, saw blades, all machinery big and small.

But there were never any instructions in your package, just the drawings and the IBM card you punched after each step was completed.

I love that type of challenge.

With my mind never stopping and always having loved tools, building plastic models and anything else I could get into, I took to this like a baby duck to water. I was able to find the sizes I needed in the scrap pile almost right away—a fact noticed by every man in the shop, as the news was out about what was happening. I can tell you they all were watching, and almost every single guy was rooting for me. I could feel it. They were walking by just waiting for me to ask them anything so they could help, like from all the way across the shop. I was nowhere near a water fountain or the coffee machine or bathroom. They were just going out of their way on their own time to see if I needed help. These were the type of men that were doing this work in 1976; it was a whole different world than today, seems like. Almost all were veterans. It's also why I've never forgotten it and why I loved so many of them so much.

Of course, the scrap had to be sheared to the right sizes, but Soto, the eleven-year shear operator, stepped aside quickly but was ready in a moment's notice to help me. I didn't want to seem too sharp or too fast, so I took my time on the cut layouts so that all could see. After a couple of approving nods all around, I cut everything very quickly and went to Randy's table. But I had no tools, and, of course, his were locked up.

Jim, the lead man, came up to me right then and said, "Come on." We went to his personal tool lockers by the office, a huge complex of tool cabinets I had never even seen open. He opened up two of them and simply said, "Use these, but lock it."

There was more than enough. I couldn't honestly say I knew what every tool in those two cabinets was even used for. I was more than impressed, I tell you.

To make it easier to lay out on cold steel, we used a highly watered-down version of the primer that was sprayed to protect the finished parts. The lines and markings you would make to define the multitude of punches, drilling, cutting, alignments, welding, etc. could then be much more easily seen. Most mechanics also used a grease pen to highlight what had been laid out with their scribe (a pencil of very sharp steel) and to make notes to themselves or for another mechanic about the process being applied. Guys developed individual ways of marking their layouts—some to the point of quite artistic.

I took my time. I could have laid something like this out in about three or four minutes, but I couldn't let anybody see me do something like that on a first test for apprenticeship.

I did a textbook layout with plenty of notes (if I would have gotten this job assigned to me three months from then, not only would I have been pretty insulted, but I certainly would not have bothered with the grease pen notes), but I knew every single guy of the twenty-three or so in the shop was watching, so I gave it to them the way they wanted to see it done. No problem.

I called Jim over to proof the layout. You were required to get your lead man to proof your layout, or inspect it, before any cutting, punching, welding, etc. were done until you made mechanic three in the shop.

He went over it like an IRS auditor does with a known tax cheater and then finally summed up, a bit perplexed. "You're off on the lines for the mounting holes by a little less than one-sixteenth of an inch. Did you miss your scribe mark?" he said while scratching his head a bit. Obviously the difficult part of the layout was perfect, and it didn't make sense to miss this easy part.

I said, "No, Jim, the bend allowance."

He said, "You're gonna punch it out flat then brake it?" (To "brake" something was to bend it to an angle.)

I said I sure was; if I went through the trouble of braking the guard first, then I would have to hand drill each one of the mounting holes. Hand drilling was surely not easy or accurate with heavy steel. It would also take at least ten minutes per hole, with a clamping hassle for the drill eight separate times! If I could punch it first as a flat piece of steel, it would be identical every time in exact location, and the whole job of getting the mounting holes perfect would take less than ten minutes total.

But you would have to allow a bend allowance to make the holes wind up in the perfect position called for in the plans when the piece was bent because steel stretches just a little bit when you bend it. They had a simple handbook for this attached on Don's front door. In my case, it called for three-sixty-fourths of an inch bend allowance.

I guess they had always bent the chain guards first when they always did them. I didn't know, but there were several looks as a half-dozen mechanics seemed to be loafing around the shears near the table I was at. Jim flipped my tape measure back to me underhanded, as the proofing was done, with some kind of look I still haven't figured out yet. He then gave me the salaam with both arms a couple of times and just walked off.

One of the mechanics at the next table simply started clapping lightly but steadily. The test was over, even though the part wasn't finished yet. I punched, final cut, bent, then welded up the finished chain guard in about another hour or so, about an hour and half to completion, from scrap. There was no more watching from anybody after Jim's inspection. I was just another mechanic on a table after a couple of hours. Show over.

But I had forgotten to punch my IBM card one single time during the building process! *How could I have forgotten that?* Don had even reminded me! So I punched all processes out at the same time, figuring that was better than no reporting. The beginning of union issue I couldn't possibly have imagined.

But my gosh, I *really had* been going as slow as I could, regardless of whether or not I was a union member. I mean, what did that matter?

Too bad that I found out later it was considered a four-and-a-half-hour job for a mechanic five grade, by negotiated agreement between the "Union" and the "Suits," the executive and engineering branch of what we called the Office.

I was promoted to apprentice mechanic the next day.

Usually, a new demand or responsibility like that would have brought on increased anxiety almost immediately. But not in this case. This was different and seemed completely natural for several reasons. I had planned to climb the ladder here; I needed more money. The main supervisor, Don, understood me, as much as anyone could at the time, and the job was quite interesting and challenging. I was sure I could take on the extra work, as being a mechanic was much more demanding than any position in the paint department, and still maintain my college ambitions.

It was quite a plateful, even though I was learning to get by on less and less sleep and had raised my caffeine intake quite a bit to help me cheat the clock even more than my adrenaline problem already did. This time the anxiety would come later, an unknown train wreck ahead, despite being quite happy in my relationship, job, and school. The combination of the three would boil up to anxiety due to time demands I was simply unable to meet or control.

* *

In October of 1976, our company got the largest ever order from Russia in the history of foreign exchange with that country, as of that date.

I can't remember the financial numbers, but the order was for fifty giant track-based, fully movable, oil-drilling platforms the likes of which had never been manufactured before. The last five of these giant rigs would be more than two hundred feet wide, five hundred fifty feet long, and have over sixteen tank-like tracks to propel them around a giant oil field in Russia. It could drill deeper than ten thousand feet. Every single guy was talking about it.

And our shop would build all the control stations, housings for electrical, plumbing, and oil control, including all instrumentation. Absolutely some of the most critical parts of the whole project.

They immediately put us on twelve-hour shifts. We had to finish every job they had already sold to get ready to start on what was already being called the "Russian job."

This was putting an unbelievable strain on not only me but my relationship with Wendy, irrespective of any other issues. I was working from 3:30 p.m. to 3:30 a.m., Monday to Friday, with an eight-hour shift from 7:30 a.m. to 3 p.m. on Saturday. I had college four days a week beginning at 9:15 a.m. I would get out of school between 1:30 and 2:30 p.m. and then head straight to work. As a result of all that, we were only able to see each other for a few hours each week on Saturday nights and Sundays and some Tuesdays. She was in junior college, kind of on hold a bit for me because she had multiple scholarships and could have gone to any college she wanted to. She just was choosing to hold herself back to my pace for me. I know that now. I really didn't realize it then.

Wow. What a catch I must have seemed like by then. Like last prize. You have to know now that love does matter.

I apprenticed in three and a half weeks, in a sixteen-week program. Don filed the papers for me to come in as a mechanic three because he snarled at me in a kind of friendly but warning way, "We can't waste Jim's time on your layouts, Clay." What could I say? My pay was almost doubling again.

The apprentice program was generally two weeks at each of eight specialty tables, learning all facets of building every style of part they built, from things like simple cabinets to highly complex machinery guards and walls for the drilling platforms.

They didn't need to apprentice me on a welding table. I had previously had my welding x-rayed for soundness while working as an assistant on the walls table with Chris. To show the whole shop Don would not play favors with me, he gave me the "stool" order for my first assignment.

The "stool" (I can't mention the real names this job was called by the mechanics) was probably the absolute worst of the jobs that went through the shop. It was very heavy, one-fourth-inch-thick steel that needed twenty punches per stool on an order of fifty stools for stock that also required one thousand brake-press operations to complete *before* the welding. To give you an idea of the welding requirement for this job, you were allowed four days to weld the stools alone. It was the worst of the jobs. I just told Jim, when he handed me the packet, "Thanks, buddy." He looked very defensive and said, "Don told me!" I had to laugh. Jim was awesome, and I just told him, "It's cool, man; no problem. Three days, and I'm done."

They had made me my own table. There had been no retirement or quitting by a mechanic to make room for me. They simply cleared out some old machinery; replaced a lot of cabinetry to the paint area that was now mysteriously clean and highly organized (I was going to have to talk to that painter three; he was doing all right there!); brought in a brand new, three-phase, very elaborate "stick" welding machine—a new welding machine we were all learning—a weld-by-wire system that would be known as MIG welding; a complete hydraulics and torch system; a new crane; three giant tool cabinets, and then Don said, "There you go; get busy." I guess it was just pure luck that it was about ten feet from Don's office or that it had its own overhead door right next to the table.

We *had* been down some of the same trails; we both knew the reason for that door so near me. Neither one of us could control our temperature, but the foreman's shop was air-conditioned. Even so, Don always kept clean shirts folded in a drawer in his desk. Later on in life I would do the same in my offices.

The overhead door wasn't as good as air-conditioning, but he was doing all he could for my sweating.

I did the stools in less than three shifts and then punched those mothers *out*. That job resulted in my one and only return in the history of my work there: I left out a hole out of one of the stools. I got a hard time for that from every single mechanic that day too: "Can we get you a job that's simpler, man?" "Can't even do the first one right, Clay?" or "Hey, Clay, I've got some punch work I need you to do; can you help me?" done as sarcastically as possible with as much profanity as they could imagine. It was really my initiation into their world. I have to tell you it made me more proud than it would ever make me mad or insulted. I knew I belonged somewhere now.

And I went to work like a madman. I was really learning how to abuse myself by using the aspects of the disease that could make me successful for my personal benefit and just trying to ignore or deny the negative parts because they didn't fit in with a perfect self-image. A perfect self-image is an important cousin of denial. A combination of ego and disease like that helped me outwork anybody, on any shift.

But it wasn't the healthy use of natural talent it appeared to be, and I knew it.

I also knew I had become a liar. A big one. And I didn't have a clue how to stop it.

# Disease in Full Bloom

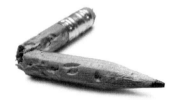

J im had been giving me some great jobs, some of which had
only been built a few times or were quite complex—
no beginner jobs ever. I was having the time of my life;
even though I was a little tired and just not feeling quite all the
way there, my work was quite good—at least I thought so. But
sometimes lately I was very sick each morning, seemed nervous
and anxious for no reason at all, and my skin itched all the time.

After my ninety days' probationary period as a mechanic
three, or apprentice mechanic, I was due for review. Either you
were left alone (usual), upgraded (rare at ninety days in this job,
as you can imagine), or sent back through the apprentice program (bad). Monthly, on the Friday that your IBM production
reviews came back, you had a private meeting with Don in his
office to review them when he handed you your paycheck. I was
called in last—no good. *B* for Ballentine usually meant I was
called in second.

When I was called into Don's office, I thought, *Uh-oh.*
*What's going on?* I knew my work was good. I just knew it. Don
seemed totally disinterested and was just looking around like a
tourist at Disneyland. There were four "suits" there in the office
too. I had *never* seen suits like these in our shop or in the Office
either for that matter. These weren't the cheap polyester suits

I had seen the engineers and office workers wear; these guys looked like real money, possibly executives.

I was sure I was done. *They've found out I lied about age or school, something. I am done. Oh God, I need this job too! Maybe I can lie my way out of this somehow.*

The youngest of the suits spoke up first. "Mr. Ballentine, we have been reviewing your production reports for the past three months since you came out of apprenticeship so fast."

I was about to jump in that I had specifically asked Jim for some of the tougher and more complex-type jobs and I was sure I could speed it up when college was done at the end of the term when he finished his thoughts. "And you have been running at an average of 340 percent, over 400 percent last month alone, of maximum possible production estimates. Can you explain that for us?"

For one of the few times—and I mean few times—in my life, I didn't have a clue what to say. I looked at Don for help, but suddenly he was very busy with something on his shoe.

I fell back on what would then become my routine lie when caught in such situations: the old everybody-deserves-credit lie. I began to tell them how each mechanic had been helping me at every stage, probably costing them their own production time losses; that we had the best and sharpest lead man in the company, who always was helping me daily; and that I had the best boss in the world in Don, who kept us all motivated and the shop in perfect order. I mean, I put it out there pretty good I thought, with some gusto too.

The oldest, and by far the best dressed of the suits, who had said nothing the entire time, just said "bull" with a kind of a disgusted look on his face and was looking me square in the eyes.

I admit, after about ten seconds, I blinked first and sort of dropped my head.

Don finally stepped in now, saying I was just a fast worker at times, that I had been working extra hard to impress him, Jim, and the gang because I had come up the ladder so quickly, and that I was a natural with a lot of different tools.

But the suits just weren't buying it. You could tell. And they weren't leaving Don's office either.

Don handed me my pay envelope and said to get back to work. The oldest suit spoke up again, very loudly and directly to me, and to me only, before I could go, "Those time estimates are just way too easy, aren't they?"

No more lying today. I was exhausted anyway. I hadn't been able to eat much for two months now, and never in the morning; plus, why bother? This guy could just see right through me like an X-ray machine. I just said, "Yes, sir, they are; a bonehead can do it in about half the time you allow." He walked over, shook my hand, and gave me what most of his associates would probably have called his smile. I wasn't sure of that look, and I shook hands with the other three and beat it out of there as fast as I could.

I found out after I left the office that the oldest guy in the nicest suit was the CEO.

The Union War had begun. I had just fired the first shot and didn't even know it.

W hen the Russian dies landed at my table by forklift early one shift, we all knew who was going to get the instrument panels. It was necessary to punch in the words on oilfield equipment; paint just won't get it done.

I wasn't going to have to learn Russian, but I was going to have to learn the Russian alphabet or one wrong punch and the whole instrument panel was ruined. Oh man, I could see this coming a mile away. So did everyone else; although there were several of a much senior grade that thought they might get a job assignment like that, there was little relative jealously among us. Many times mechanics had to work together, several guys at once on one project just to get the assignment done.

I left the office to find the new model Russian instrument panels work order on my table. A completely different work order than the routine instrument panels every apprentice had to complete. I swear everything looked like Kaopectate!

Oh boy. What a day!

I did ruin four of the order of twenty-five, so I had to build twenty-nine. I have to tell you that I have been able to pick up Spanish, French, and Italian languages quickly and travel using them somewhat comfortably with the occasional mistake. But when the entire alphabet is different, it's just a whole new ball game.

You can pretty easily pick up and repeat without mistake the few obvious ones for *oil pressure, RPMs,* and *hydraulic pressure,* but it was the toughest job I have ever had in building or construction. It really took every ounce of concentration I had for the entire three-day period to do those.

Friends, did I hear it from *every* mechanic when I had to throw out four boards for incorrect wording. On one of them, it was the very last instrument description to be done! I was so frustrated with that one that I had to go outside for about fifteen minutes just to cool off. My anxiety wouldn't allow me to make mistakes, any mistakes, without confusing my self-worth with the error. This would result in more anger at myself and consequently more anxiety. As the disease would grow, it would take longer and longer time or time-outs for me to get over issues that simply weren't that important. A routine mistake had been and still was taken personally by me, and I was physically pushed by my thyroid disease into exaggerated behavior patterns. For years this had been anger. Anger either at myself, someone specific I felt was at blame for the issue, but I had much less ability to control the anger now. Sometimes I would just lash out at anyone who happened to be handy. When that happened, many times within an hour or so, I would feel worse than ever, embarrassed by both my loss of control and the pain I had caused somebody needlessly. A cycle you can easily understand that would grow and grow and grow.

When I came back in from cooling off outside, the mechanics blasted me with insults, and their vocabulary was expanding now to include *Russian* profanity! These guys gave it to me nonstop for three days while I built them. Honestly, I had to laugh an awful lot myself about it as well, partially because I knew they were a just a bit jealous too.

I saw Don watching me move the finished twenty-five completed panels to the grinders (the workers that smooth off all the rough edges of the metal before it's primed). It had been about three days to do the panels since the suits, including the CEO, had been in. As I headed over to the time station to punch the job out, he was waiting for me at the IBM clock and said, "Punch out and then come in." To "come in" meant to come straight to his office.

When I walked in and said my usual, "What's up, chief?" (I was in a great mood after finishing those panels and just more than pleased to be done with that!), he said, "We're changing your grade to mechanic ten X, effective tonight."

I knew that sounded good but had never heard of it. I knew you could go up to mechanic fifteen, which was the highest manufacturing grade you could have; the next step was lead man and ultimately foreman, but I had never heard of *X*.

"Ten X?" I asked him.

"It means you'll only build *firsts*" (the term in manufacturing shops for the first or prototype unit built). And then he almost growled at me, "And the *X* means you're off the IBM clock. You will not punch that clock again until I tell you; do you hear me?"

*Okay, okay; good grief.* But it bugged me a bit right in the craw. I had just been busting my butt with everything I had for that panel order. I was getting another promotion, but it seemed like he was jumping my buns at the same time. I just didn't get it and told him so straight up.

He went cooler and relaxed a bit, asked me to sit down, then quietly told me, "There's a union problem—with time per job now, every single job we do on existing rigs, and also you'd better know those panels you just finished were scheduled for fifteen days."

T he camaraderie was breaking up. There's no other way to say it. Certainly the nonstop sixty- to sixty-eight-hour weeks of grueling physical work to tight tolerances with no mistakes were part of the problem. But the shop steward, Randy—the man whose table I had used to pass my first test for apprenticeship and had never failed to show or help me with something new—had begun to completely avoid me. Several others in the shop, who were also union members, were giving me the cold shoulder.

And I was the problem.

My anxiety and disease were acting up again and had grown now to include bowel irritability. I just lied about this to myself and Wendy by saying that the roach coach (the food trucks that go around to manufacturing and construction sites to sell food and drink) food was killing me, then laughing it off and changing the subject quickly. I was still sweating more than anybody I knew ever did and way more than I thought I should, but I knew it cleared my pores, so why worry? My joints had begun to hurt a little bit from time to time, but I simply thought with all the extra workload we had had that would be natural.

All of these were absolutely perfect rationalizations. If you're having some of these same problems, you can make the same ones to yourself right now; it's easy. I know. It did it for more than forty years myself.

Unfortunately, they're also the signs of disease—many different and serious diseases in fact.

I needed a doctor right then, and so did my boss, Don, but neither of us knew it or probably would have admitted to it.

Besides, one of the medical instruments, vital to detect some of our problems, wouldn't be invented for almost twenty-five more years.

●　●

Of course, with the first "first" work order for the instrument panels completed way earlier than planned, they had no other drawings ready for me to go to work on. So I was forced to spend the next two and a half shifts helping Chris build walls. Chris wasn't a union member, and if he had been, he could have cared less about what was going on. He was a very good mechanic, could work anywhere in the world, and had the confidence to know it. He tried to get me to laugh about the events that occurred several times, but I just never quite had his sense of humor, especially about what was happening in the shop. Chris was simply the kind of guy that was best friend to about twenty guys.

I had never approached what I was doing as a sheet-metal mechanic conducting a job. Rather, I saw this as a giant puzzle book, just like the kinds I had done all my life as a kid in those comic book-sized magazines. Only quite a bit better than that really. You always got new puzzles (especially after you had been there a year or more), were completely free to build it the way you wanted, and you could take a lot of pride out of creating some of the products we built from flat pieces of steel. I never came to work anywhere near late; the truth was that I couldn't wait to go to work. It was just going to be another new set of puzzle books.

At least until the Union thing began and then just wouldn't seem to die.

Also unfortunately, at this point in time, I was going to have to add sleep disorder to my constant medical symptoms list. Although, I would lie about this problem to my girlfriend, her parents, my future wife, all the friends and family I've ever had since I was nineteen years old, as well as every doctor I saw for more than thirty years.

Never a particularly good sleeper, now, even when exhausted after a twelve-hour shift, I could not nap before classes or sleep much at all on my school day off or Sundays. Many hyperthyroid sufferers have a lot of trouble sleeping, especially when they encounter what most would call routine stress. This may cause a hyperthyroidic to either "leak," as in my case, or overproduce adrenaline at an even higher level than their diseased condition routinely causes. This in turn will physically prohibit just resting, much less sleeping. Counting sheep or using self-relaxation techniques does absolutely nothing for those who are hyperthyroid; it's a glandular problem, not a mental one. I was already routinely into denial and now rationalizing this as overwork (I guess you can add diagnosing myself as another huge ego flaw and complete lack of facing reality). At least I had two weeks' paid vacation coming, as I had been there a year.

But the truth is, for the first time ever in my career there, I began to contemplate quitting instead of vacationing. I never wound up taking the vacation. I just had them pay me the two weeks' extra instead.

●　●

Finally a new set of plans for the new model rig were ready. The operator's cabin of the instrument panels I had just completed. The cabin was three-sided with windows and doors on both sides, a large front window, and an open rear leading directly to the rigging machinery right behind the operator or driller and the driving controls for the rig in a completely separate compartment near the front of the rig. These were commonly built in our shop, called "OCs," but the new rigs were more than twice the size of our standard rigs, and the Russian operator cabin had to grow a bit and be redesigned.

I saw the plans and two pallets of flats (precision-cut flat steel waiting to be hand built) at my table when I came to shift. I looked the drawings over very carefully, checked a couple of Soto's cuts, and then went up to Chris's table to help him finish some long twelve-foot panel welds.

Jim, the lead man, came by about thirty minutes into the shift and said, "Are you about done here? They finally got a job out for you. Didn't you see it at your table?"

I told him we were virtually through, but it didn't matter. I also told him I had reviewed the drawings for the new OCs and they couldn't be built, or rather, they shouldn't be built the way they were drawn.

He just stared at me a second, rubbed on his chin the way he always did when he was in thought, then said, "When you finish here, get the plans, and let's meet in Don's office." I said sure, about a half hour or so I thought, and looked to Chris; he nodded his approval.

It was less than that to finish. I grabbed the plans and knocked on Don's door. Jim was already inside. Don spoke up immediately, "What's wrong with the new OC?"

"Where do you want me to start?" was kind of the snidely worded comeback I should have saved for the engineers, not Don, but he knew what I meant and didn't take offense. After all, he didn't draw this trash up.

"Why not at the beginning then?" he said.

"The two lateral sides are cut longer than the front cabin plate; unless we build a special platform, with steps, you couldn't even place the OC on a flat piece of steel. It would rock back and forth like one of those chairs you get at cheap restaurants that has one leg shorter than the other!"

He almost jumped out of his chair to look at the plans I had in my hand. Such a mistake would be unheard of in the company we worked for. Cabins had flanges with one-inch bolts along the base where they attached to a rig; then those bolts were welded over. An OC had to fit perfectly flush with the deck of the rig or it was junk—forget how unsafe it would be. We unrolled the plans on his drafting table, and I showed him the measurements. I hadn't bothered to check all the shear cuts that Soto had made because he didn't get a copy of the plans, only a shear list, and I can guarantee that steel was cut to the proper length they had called for. It just wouldn't work.

"Second, Don, look at the doors and handles. They're all set up wrong and for left handers." The door handles had been designed to push in the lock button, pull up, and then pull the door out to enter, with the handle facing to the left. Exactly the opposite of every door we'd ever built and opposite the way almost every car was built too. This was a very difficult way to use a door, especially when you're covered in grease and oil and had heavy gloves on as these drillers did *and* were climbing a small stepladder just to enter. The opposite side was exactly wrong, in the exact proportion. Somebody just drew the handles up and put them upside down on the wrong side. Period.

Don moaned and let out a long sigh; even Jim turned around and sat down after that.

"Don, that's not all by a long shot. Look. The door measurements don't add up; the hole opening is four and one-fourth inches wider than the door. Even with a giant hinge, the door couldn't be made to shut because the door locking bolt is only one inch long, and there's gonna be a draft all the way around too!" No amount of weather stripping was going to cover up that kind of gap, especially when it was all the way around.

"There're a couple of minor things I saw too. The window opening is bigger than the window sizing, but that can be fixed by just ordering larger glass, but somebody's got to tell them before they order 'em. Several of the corners won't miter 'cause there're no bend allowances, so we'll be short with gaps all the way around, but I could weld some of that out. I stopped looking them over when I saw all this, so I don't know if that's all or not."

Don made several notes and then noted to us a few additional things he saw that were wrong and told me to wait at my table. We probably needed to recut the job on several items and do some adjustments. He asked if I would mind helping Soto with that this shift. I said, "Of course not. You just let me know. No problem, chief."

Don emerged from his office just a couple of minutes later. "The office is coming down." That meant the engineers assigned to this drawing would be coming to the shop to *discuss* their drawings with us.

I had a bad feeling about this. In the year and one month I had worked there, I had never heard of engineer suits coming down to the shop, especially to *discuss* anything. The engineers were near the top of the Suits food chain, right under executives. High-level engineers don't visit any of the manufacturing shops. That was for their subordinate entry level draftsmen to do. The shops were hot, dirty, noisy places, with constantly flashing welding that could temporarily blind you going on all the time. Obviously dangerous places, every shop had, huge machinery making ear-busting rhythmic noises as they cut, sheared, or stamped raw steel, and enormous parts moving around overhead by crane all the time. The shops were considered by the suits and all the office workers on a par roughly just a notch or two above hell.

Strange, when I think back and write this to you, it seemed just like home to me.

Anyway, we could see them coming down the dirt road that led to our sheet metal shop, pissed their shoes were getting dirty, wearing those late 1970s polyester dress shirts, cheap ties, with a pen and slide rule shield in their shirt pockets. They looked just like some of the characters in the movie that would come out later called *Nerds*. I swear. I almost broke out laughing before they even got to the shop. You could see the anger in their faces.

Don called me back in after they arrived.

The two engineers, one who was the designer and the other, a senior grade engineer, was the checker, headed straight for Don's office. Jim came out and told me to "go right in." When I walked back into Don's office, these guys looked at me, my dirty work overalls, bags under my eyes, hair in a mess from wearing the welding helmet to help Chris earlier, my young age (nineteen), sweating like crazy, and gave me a look like they had just stepped in a really nasty pile of smelly dog feces.

Don recognized it and started to get mad. I could see he was also starting to get red in the face and neck. I was a little insulted too, but my ego was much smaller on the job for some reason at that time. *Who cares?* I thought.

He said, "Gentlemen, this is Clay Ballentine, Ten X mechanic, the only one in the company. He, and only he, will build your prototypes, and the executives have taken him completely off the IBM clock. Got it?"

They didn't like it, not one single bit. They had wanted somebody's job for making them come to the shop. I bet they had even said something like that around their offices before they stomped out. Now it looked like they were really stuck with me because I could guarantee you they wouldn't go to the suits about these crummy drawings, much less a mechanic who rightly called them out about it or his boss.

But they did not speak to me or acknowledge me or my presence the rest of the meeting.

They physically turned away from me and then turned sharply on Don and demanded, "Where is the list you have made of the things that are wrong?" Don handed them a copy of the legal pad-sized long list we had made just an hour before. Now I started to get mad. You don't turn like that on the most respected foreman in the company (and also my friend) like you are some kind of royalty or something! I had seen the CEO himself in that office, and he certainly never conducted himself like that. So I started to ask them, "Hey, could you give being a jerk a thirty-minute break for us?" or something like that when Don physically moved one of them aside with his arm rather sharply to get right up in my face before I could finish because by now I was moving toward them aggressively.

I honestly hadn't realized it until Don and I talked about it later that shift. I had almost lost it again, but he stopped it.

Don said, with a pretty serious look right in my face, "Wait for me at your table; help Lonnie if he needs it." Lonnie was rolling giant flats into hydraulic drums, and mechanics needed help for that, even with a crane. I took over for the painter who was helping him and waited for Don.

The engineers came out after less than ten minutes and stomped back to the office on the hill.

Don did not come out for almost twenty more minutes. And there was a problem.

Have you ever seen somebody get beet red when they get mad? I mean they have a real red-color flush all over the visible parts (and most of the nonvisible parts too) of their face, ears, and neck—arms too if you can see them. Their eyes will bulge out some, they will have a harsh breathing sound, and they won't be able to talk rationally for a second. They may have some other issues going on at that exact time too. Some you will see; some you can't. Think back because you have seen this, maybe several times. This is probably not just somebody with a bad temper or a temper problem; this is somebody with a medical problem, and it could be a fairly serious or life-threatening medical problem.

It takes one to know one. I knew he needed some help right then, and it was my job. I caused this.

I walked over to him, and he was *boiling* mad as they say, in a burst of color change, both eyes were bulging a little, his right side was trembling, both right arm and right leg just a tiny bit, as were his lips. He did not speak to me as I approached; he couldn't. He was in what my personal experiences over the years have made me call that time of a *burst* as the "it's-taking-every-thing-I've-got-to-control-myself-I-can't-talk-now" syndrome.

I've learned that the medical term for this condition is "thyroid blush." This health phenomenon occurs to many of us with thyroid disease when we're hit with major stress or anger. In a few years, it would begin to happen to me as well then grow in ferocity and frequency as my disease progressed.

I walked over to him and by complete luck and accident decided to try something with no idea what would happen. I put my arm around him like you would a male buddy you're going to tell something really private to, and I could feel he was in a complete sweat, and it was a cold sweat. I acted and sounded, with a whispered voice, like I was telling him a very deep and dark secret and spoke very softly in his ear, "Lonnie just gave me three points and the Cowboys! Can you believe it, man?"

It definitely worked.

Don was a huge Dallas Cowboys fan. The game was a home game at Texas Stadium, and the Cowboys were a ten-point favorite that week on Monday night. The painters had rigged a radio setup so we could get the ABC radio broadcast of the game throughout the shop that would start in just about an hour or so. Now Lonnie would not have given me three points and the Cowboys if his life depended upon it—*nobody* would have—but that lie didn't matter, especially then. In fact, in my experiences, the bigger the whopper of a story, the faster the change may occur in your friend, especially if you can cause a laugh.

You don't have to know them that well either. Don't use that excuse to not help them. You can come up with a whopper of some interest to anybody you know casually.

Don began to relax immediately. I'm not a doctor or psychologist. I don't even have a college degree, but like I said, it takes one to know one, and I simply got lucky. I think it's the total changing of the subject that causes someone with thyroid disease, especially someone interested in what your "privacy" message is to them, to stop their brain a second, process the new question about a private, pleasant, and different subject, and develop a response to something that's not related to what's been a trigger to an extreme anxiety/thyroid/adrenal/hormonal burst event. This buys time for our systems to recover, just a bit maybe, but enough a lot of the time.

I hope that I've explained this well, and I know it's not scientific, but try it when you see it if something like this happens to somebody you work with or care about. It has been almost 100 percent successful every single time for me, and I have been doing this for thirty-two years since that night—sometimes for complete strangers!

We talked for a good ten minutes about the Dallas defense, especially the defensive line and if they could get sacks, the Dallas running game, and what kind of advantage we would have on our home turf instead of the grass field like they had at the Redskins' home field. All kinds of game stuff while we walked very slowly away from the rolling machine to my table area. Jim later told me nobody even looked up or spoke usually when Don got this way. *Don got this way a lot before?* I had never seen it in a year.

I guess Don had gotten pretty good at hiding his problems too.

Within a minute or two he dropped almost to a normal color hue, the trembling stopped, and he shivered a bit while standing in front of the overhead door at my table (always open, winter or summer) because his sweating had stopped and a cold wet shirt will give you the shivers (I should know). I pulled the door down, slipped the drawings from his left hand, and tried to slide them under my table.

That brought him back. He was back to business but a much different man now.

He simply told me then, with some measure of emotion in his voice and eyes, almost tears, "Build this just exactly like they've drawn it, not one change; hear me?"

I just said, "No problem, chief. Consider it done."

 •  •

When I finished the operator's cabin, I think the best way to describe what this thing looked like was if Timothy Leary, on his best LSD, would have designed an operator's cabin, it would have looked like this one did.

Jim was almost living at my table, constantly checking my measurements to make sure they conformed; by now he had almost rubbed his chin raw. Don was coming out to check all the time too. From day one of construction, it looked like a monstrosity.

The whole shop had grown much quieter as I built this "thing." In a sense, like the actors would say in some of those Indian or war movies, "I don't like it. It's too quiet out there." Everybody knew there was going to be hell to pay coming for the days of work and use of expensive one-fourth-inch-thick cold steel for something like this junk was. But I was merrily working away with little concern for that stuff. I'd gotten my hands full just trying to solve the construction problems because so few of the measurements fit.

I tell you, I learned some new tricks on that one, but I got it done—five full shifts to get one cabin completed, and I was going to crane it back to the grinders when Don beat me to it. He told Jim to call the grinders up. We weren't going to move this *anywhere* until inspection. Both our grinders came up to begin cleaning up all the welds (there were many places where I had had to just fill in with welding rods and stick weld-up holes where the steel simply did not meet up), and the grinders went to work really hard on those areas first because they showed glaring design problems. But Don said, "No!" as they leaned into it. "Just clean the burrs off." The chief inspector for the company and the lead inspector for the machine shop, also friends of Don's, got there about thirty minutes later, before the grinders were even through. Don told the grinders, "Good enough." And they seemed relieved to be going back to their regular station.

The machinist inspector had a huge case with him with precision calipers to eight feet long. Between these two guys, this project was going to get the inspection of its life from the very best inspectors in the company. I was kind of nervous, but I knew it was right; it had been checked by Don and Jim a thousand times. But I was still a little nervous.

When they arrived at my table and looked at the cabin, they gave Don a look like "What, are you kidding us?" But Don was all business they could tell, cracked no smiles or funny stories, and simply said, "Tight tolerance check." He handed them the drawings.

They went to work. They never said anything, to us or each other. In about twenty-five minutes, they took their grease pens and put a huge check mark on the cabin, both of them did, each with their different initials. The chief inspector also added his own okay to it. They left, shaking their heads.

I asked Don if he wanted me to crane it back to the grinders to finish. He said, "No, I've got other plans." Our shift was almost over, and I helped Chris for less than an hour until the whistle blew. There wasn't a new set of drawings yet for me to work on. The order was for five cabins but had been altered to one after the confrontation with the engineers.

The next day I arrived at my shift about thirty minutes early, pretty standard for me. There was a crowd of workers near the main overhead door to the shop, the one closest and within view of the office. There were guys on forklifts from the shipping department, men and women shift leaders on bicycles (they used them to get around the huge complex of about a hundred acres easier), and just workers of all kinds who were either coming on or off shift assembled in front of the sheet metal shop in mass. They were staring up at the cabin I'd built, which had by now been hung on wires in the open doorway for all to see and admire. It reminded me of the old horror and western movies we've all seen where a disfigured body had been left hanging on its death noose like a grim reminder for all to observe.

There was more than just laughing and profanity; it was outright jeering from the whole hourly grade. Literally, hundreds of men and women had seen that piece of junk hung up. And the okay and check marks were clearly visible for all as well.

I just thought, *Oh no!*

Don was just outside his door but waiting for me when I walked toward my table. Most of the first shift was still cleaning up. He had his hands on his hips, feet spread, I remember, a little like a gunfighter might look.

He said, "I'm going to call them. Want to come in?"

I said, "No, Don. No offense, but not especially."

He said, "Okay, see you," and headed straight back inside his office.

About twenty minutes later, we could see them coming back down the dirt road, but this time, there were four men, and one of the men was much older. They stopped about fifty feet outside the shop and looked up. They looked for a while and then walked back to the office. They did not come inside or speak with anyone from the shop.

Both Chris and I saw with perfect clarity what had happened, but the way we were welding up walls when Jim came around, you would have thought we were blind. Jim came up and patted me on the back lightly. "Don wants you in his office when you have a minute."

I had a minute right then.

When I entered Don's office, he was leaned back in his chair and had the smile of the cat that ate the canary, which, in the world of business, I guess he just had. I was really glad, even though I had been very nervous and had almost gotten sick at my stomach when I walked up to our shop door and saw the cabin hung up like that. That was almost a declaration of total war act.

Don simply said, "The suits have asked you to make the changes on any plans you get on paper first then send them back to engineering for approval before you would begin to rebuild it to your specs. Is that okay with you, sweetheart?"

Whew. I let out some air and just said, "Great. No problem, chief!"

I decided to quit this great job that night after my shift. It appeared there was no other option. I had to admit to myself I was just out of gas, my grades were dropping in school, and I felt I was losing touch with Wendy too. I had a bit of cash saved up, this term's tuition paid, many skills I could do part time, but mostly, I thought this job was making me pretty sick.

I guess I've got to admit that in very late 1977, just after I turned twenty years old, I was already nauseous in the mornings and large parts of the day. I had joint pain, could not sleep well, had almost uncontrollable sweating, shivering at times with cold feet, and sometimes really dry skin, and occasional nagging anger about very small things that I knew meant nothing. I went through thirty-one years of increasing symptoms and more and more denial before I would finally admit any of this to anyone, including myself. But even then, only at the cost of an incredibly traumatic and potentially fatal health emergency at the age of fifty-one.

When you look up *hardheaded* in the dictionary, my picture is right there.

And throughout most of this book so far, I bet you've thought I seem like a reasonably intelligent person. But the real truth is I was a bigger idiot than anybody has ever known. And in complete denial to boot.

I also had not made the connection yet that my mom had, and was having, virtually the exact same set of problems.

And … why was I so, so … anxious?

W hen I asked Don for a couple of minutes in his office near the end of the shift, I got a worried look right away from him. This was not the way Clay acted.

When we went in, I told him the hours and school were killing me. I was holding up the most important thing in my life, in fact, the only thing I really loved, from going on with her life and education and felt it wouldn't be long until I lost her for that alone. I never wanted to have split the shop up the way I accidentally had, and now it looked like war with the office for him as well. I was giving my two weeks' notice, and I wanted to count on a good reference from him. I also wanted him to know he had been better to me than my own father.

He did not act the least surprised, and that kind of hurt and shocked me a bit. He simply said, "Don't do this tonight. Can you meet me in the hiring office tomorrow at 2:30?" That was an hour before my shift, but I could do it as I had no classes that day. I said yes.

He said, "Thanks. I think you'll be glad you did."

T hey offered me an offshore rig job that would train out as a diver. It meant I could work a full summer offshore and earn enough money for full-time college and an apartment for the whole year. I could then do some light part-time work during the year for them to tide me over. I thought it was the greatest blessing I had ever been given. The word was not even out our company was going to participate in a large partnership of oil companies drilling along the Gulf Coast based out of Corpus Christi, Texas. It wouldn't be announced for two days yet. There were legal documents involved. It was a two-summer contract. I signed them without reading them. Don and I shook hands as we left.

There was one condition: I had to stay until several important prototypes were built out, or until March 1, 1978. I was cool with that.

Trouble was, Wendy and her parents weren't cool with that one bit. Offshore oil rig work in 1977 was very, very dangerous work, and they spent hours telling me so. But it didn't matter. I had already signed up, and couldn't they see that this was the solution?

No, they sure couldn't, and they all wanted some answers. Some straight answers.

Frankly, they had some coming, but I was too deep in my lies and denial to give them any truth now. This is the impossible corner you will eventually find yourself in when you constantly cover up and/or lie that something's wrong with you.

Where were my parents in all this, and why the heck weren't they shooting this down too? Why was I working ten months straight now of twelve-hour days plus an eight-hour Saturday shift when this was supposed to be a summer job till Wendy and I went to school together full time almost a year ago?

I lied like hell, but I was losing totally until I told them I would quit. Two days later, I gave them a cover company of a new job I had gone to that I thought I could use because I knew the receptionist really well. She wasn't there when Wendy called though, and I was really caught. Nobody by that name worked there, she was told, and it was over. The straw that broke a relationship's back. I told her it wasn't another woman or anything ridiculous like that, but I *was* going to the coast in a couple of months and wasn't quitting.

She said best of luck; she was through waiting and thought I would kill myself to boot. I told her she was due the best in life and I hoped she got it in everything. I also told her I obviously wasn't the one that could give it to her.

And it was over just that quickly. I had nothing left for me in Dallas. Might as well die on an oil rig as anyplace else. What did it matter anyway?

Add depression to the rapidly growing symptoms list now.

●   ●

I was scared to death driving to dive school.

Anxious isn't the word; petrified is probably a better analogy. But I wasn't going to quit before I arrived. Anyway, I was alone again, and I desperately needed the money.

Despite my fears, the dive school in Corpus Christi, Texas, was a great one. Almost all training went on indoors with warmer water temperature and lighter suits and boots. I got my certification and found myself on a rig, ready to actually begin construction less than three weeks after arrival.

Prior to the finish of dive school, trainees were given a complete and thorough physical. I began to admit to some of the problems I was having with the doctor. Morning nausea and occasional inability to control my temperature being two specific issues I brought to their attention as matters of health importance. They took additional X-rays and another blood sample; then I was promptly pronounced perfectly healthy.

I immediately attracted another friend, mentor, and guardian angel: Ian.

Ian was head of what the crew loosely called the "Irish Gang." At that time, many of the most experienced divers in the world were from the UK, Scotland, and both the Republic of Ireland and Ulster (Northern Ireland). They were very experienced in working at much deeper levels than our approximately seventy-three feet of water and were going to "train around" our crews. They considered our warm Gulf water and relatively shallow depths really easy work, but it wasn't, believe me.

It was my blessing that I became the "Kid" in the gang and had that name sewn on my uniforms instead of Clay.

On my ninth career-working dive, a freak storm occurred, which also developed a vicious undertow. All three divers down were injured due to unfinished cabling, myself included. So on my thirty-ninth day of offshore oil rig construction, I was involved in a near-fatal accident.

I was told Ian, just out of decompression himself after a four-hour shift at the bottom, went over the side in a perfect swan dive, from the low-level rig platform base. They said he went over like Tarzan, with an emergency air cylinder in each hand and a long piece of rope in his mouth. Only goggles and flippers, no scuba tank or wetsuit. He knew he couldn't get low enough, fast enough, with a tank, and the minutes it would take to go down the ladders to the water line would be the difference between life and death.

The only problem with going off the side like that was that particular rig deck was almost forty-five feet above the normal water line, and we were near a low tide. Ian got rewarded for his coming to our rescue and saving our lives with a major concussion and virtually every capillary broken in his face and sinuses. He was unable to dive again for over a week and had to spend a night in the hospital with all of us in decompression. All divers survived. I wound up with minor nitrogen narcosis, or "the bends."

Ian was a born hero. He died a born hero only nine months after his heroic acts on all our behalves in the Gulf in a famous North Sea oil rig explosion. I know he died trying to save others, but only a few lived. Ian was not one who survived.

Some new conditions had developed while working off-shore. I was losing my body hair. I had lost almost all the hair off my back, upper legs, and upper arms. I didn't understand this and blamed it on the constant use of the dive suits and constant decompression that was required. It's a no-brainer tip to any of today's doctors that there may be a thyroid problem.

Another new symptom I began to experience for the first time while working offshore was waking up with a sore right shoulder at times. Called "frozen shoulder" by doctors after research over the last fifteen years has revealed this as a routine symptom of untreated thyroid disease, I just felt it was due to my baseball years starting to show up after extremely physical work. I had no idea this is a dead-ringer clue for thyroid disease, one of the few that can really help a physician get the diagnosis right immediately. It's unfortunate that research appears to show that this symptom only begins to evidence itself long after the disease has fully developed in the sufferer. It's also believed a sign that additional internal body damage is, and has been, occurring.

The last health issue that developed during the time I worked offshore was a nuisance at first, ultimately turning into a serious misdiagnosis. Suddenly I developed leaking sinuses. Common for divers, especially scuba divers, are nosebleeds, but a constantly runny nose had never been a symptom I'd had before I went to work offshore or during dive training. I blamed it at first on the accident. Ultimately after seeing many doctors about it, it was always misdiagnosed as allergies. In reality, it's a sign of sinus disease where a sufferer has "burned out" some or most of the capillary tubes in their sinuses, many times the cause being excess adrenaline due to hyperthyroidism.

And my disease was in full bloom. It just wasn't diagnosed yet.

Before I even came out of decompression, in my mind, I had already quit the rig business. I was simply scared to dive again.

I would not even scuba for almost fifteen years until my loving wife helped me get over it by buying us both a scuba class together. We don't scuba regularly at all, but I am not afraid now either.

That's plenty good enough.

When I notified the rig boss I would not return to dive or build again because it was just not for me, he understood completely, and so did the gang. They were great on my last night out, and we had a cake with wine to celebrate everybody living through it.

The company understood me voiding the contract due to an accident. They didn't want to be sued, and you just didn't do that type of thing in 1978. To be short, I knew the job was dangerous when I took it.

But I had to do something else now. I didn't ever want to have any more celebrations for "living through it" in my career.

Ultimately, it was the best decision I would make to that date in my life. Unfortunately, the gang all stayed professional divers. (They would have *never* quit.) And none of the five of the best friends that a man could ever have lived two and a half years more.

I never had the money to attend any of their funerals. We had all kept in touch for the whole time, but every time one died, I couldn't even afford a plane ticket. The sadness of that has not left me for thirty-one years now. I don't expect it ever will.

I think about Ian and the gang a lot when I visit places like Hoover Dam, the Brooklyn Bridge, or see the rigs in the ocean. Men and women did really give their lives for these achievements. It is much more emotional to you when you have been so close to it like I have, but sometimes so difficult to express to others, maybe even to yourself. I have talked to many people who experienced the same sort of emotions when they visited Pearl Harbor and/or Normandy. You may have had these same type of feelings too.

If you ever have, you'll understand. Ian and the gang are a part of my life that will never go away.

●  ●

As the trauma of the diving accident began to subside, so did the sinus symptoms. But the never-ending puzzle of the inexorable ebb and flow of medical issues, with many cases of symptoms subsiding substantially before I could get a doctor's appointment, continued to plague me day after day. Within a few months, I believed the allergy diagnosis to be another "idiot mistake" by poor doctors, and I discontinued the medications for a few years until another serious misdiagnosis by an allergy specialist. The sinus problems never really went away but subsided enough at times to allow me easy rationalization and denial. This behavior flaw was made even more convenient later in my life. Ultimately, I would move to and live for more than twenty-five years before diagnosis in an area known for extreme allergy incidence, "cedar fever" in particular.

As I look back on this, I wonder, and medical science can't tell me positively one way or another, if my thyroid disease had developed to the point of what I simply term *symptom rotation*—one symptom (sometimes one I'd had before, sometimes a new one) not ever going entirely away and staying away. I would wind up treating the current symptom of major importance with medication of some sort or allowing my body's own defenses to fight it off to the point of toleration, only to find another side effect of the disease worsening to the point where the latest problem took first priority due to its recent severity.

It was just like the little Dutch boy putting his fingers in the leaking dike. Only I was running out of fingers, and new leaks were always developing.

While more and more symptoms occurring to someone with an undiagnosed disease is easy to understand, the ebb and flow of symptom severity in many thyroid disease sufferers is not scientifically understood today. I honestly believe it's highly correlated with stress, an opinion shared by many physicians around the world, including my own. Just keep in mind as of this writing, this is opinion born of experience, not a medical fact.

Theories and denial aside, the undeniable fact was my health was simply getting worse and worse.

I was on my way back to Dallas, and I was a very different person now. You probably could expect some feelings in your life to change after such an experience, but this was different. I had to make a life change. A big one.

I had been dealt some mixed-blessing lemons in my life: the overactivity, the limitless energy, the always-active mind. I felt strongly I needed to make some lemonade with all these flaws. It seemed to me like business was where I needed to go.

I also wasn't going to concentrate so much on school now. I knew my dad had made a fortune with very little education, so I believed I could too. I would never be that serious again about college. I began a different life tactic now, one I would use for the next thirty-one years.

I was going to focus on making money. A lot of it. At least a million.

And I'd stomp on anything or anybody who got in the way.

Disease ruled the body now, not the mind or the heart. The genesis was complete.

# The Ultimate in
# Self-Abuse:

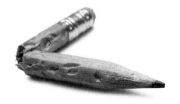

## *Using Your Disease to Make Money*

I got the lead on my first new career job while working occasional freight-car unloading for Mrs. Baird's Breads. Usually, working for the bread and pastry maker was a job reserved for the SMU athletes; Mrs. Baird's was located only a mile or so in Dallas from the Southern Methodist University campus. But it seemed like lately, at least to the foreman, that as their team's records improved, the number of workers disappeared.

I had come back from the coast without a lot of cash and had prepaid my next term's tuition, so I was short on money and working for a temporary agency while trying to find a permanent opportunity at someplace I was placed temporarily. But I was more than glad for the weekend and evening work too.

Mrs. Baird's paid well—in fact, great—and paid in cash plus a free run on their bakery rejects. Their union agreements prevented a full-time employee from entering a rail car, so the most their employees would do was drive a forklift up to the edge of the rail cars. The rail cars were loaded with eighty-pound sacks of all kinds of flour. Flour for bread, pastries, meal, and sugar.

All loaded and unloaded the same way—by hand—in eighty-pound sacks.

That was no problem for me. The foreman usually planned on four men per carload, but I told him I had a friend and that we could do it as two for the price of three. He said deal but wound up paying us as four anyway. He was just one prince of a guy.

At this time, Mrs. Baird's was still a family-owned company, and one of the grandsons, Vernon I believe his name was, regularly ran the operation day to day on the baking floor. He was a great gentleman, and working there was always a delight. They would let us come at night because in the summer the freight cars were unbearably hot. So for almost a full year, one to three nights a week, Jeff (my new roommate) and I unloaded freight cars for a few hours, got paid in cash, and got to go through the reject barrel.

The "reject barrel" was all the items—bread, pastries, fried pies, cupcakes, everything—that had failed a quality control inspection. Usually the only thing wrong was the packaging or something got smashed up or torn open, something very small was not perfect (and Mrs. Baird's did *not* send out something that was not perfect), but there was no effect at all on taste or edibility.

We got to grab all we could carry from the reject barrel after an unload. Sometimes Jeff and I would actually wear a coat, even in July and August, so we could carry out more stuff! The foreman and Mr. Vernon just laughed when they saw that; so did the whole union crew.

Mr. Vernon knew I loved the apple fried pies. That was my favorite thing they made. So after we had been working there a few months and he came to know us by sight, after we unloaded and came in for the goodies, he would order an inspection, when he saw me, of the fried pie line.

I would not go inside, even though I was finished and waiting to get paid, until they started those apple pies. I didn't care if I had to wait an hour or more, I was waiting.

To do an inspection, they had a drop-down bar to divert the line off from final packaging to check any product, usually in their labs, but also a complete visual and taste test. So when those apple pies were running, I would show up, rather sheepishly, until Mr. Vernon saw me. I knew pretty soon he would come by and order a line inspection.

That meant the operator then would immediately drop the diversion bar, and apple fried pies would coming flying off the line on a separate conveyor for an inspection. Of course, I knew by then where to stand to catch them. A dozen or more would come flying off in about five seconds, and Mr. Vernon would say, "Good enough." The bar would be pulled back up, and the pies went down the line again. I went home with several meals, time after time.

God bless them all there.

Mrs. Baird's and Mr. Vernon didn't know they kept Jeff and me from going hungry a lot.

Jeff and I were a lot alike with the overenergy issue, only his had come from a serious brain injury in a car wreck in Arkansas. Jeff had nearly died during that wreck when he was thrown from his pickup truck. It left him with an energy problem, as well as occasional depression and moodiness.

As I look back at it, I understand now that your thyroid can be greatly affected by head injuries, just like any other part of your body can. Thyroid disease symptoms also mimic many of the symptoms of head and brain trauma. So it turned out we sort of were two peas in a pod; his due to a head injury, and mine due to an as of yet undiagnosed thyroid disease.

Either way, we were great comfort to each other.

We lived in some very rough apartments across the street from a housing project in a very suspect part of Dallas. But it was cheap, right in the middle of town, and all utilities were paid. I knew I wouldn't be living there for long. I just needed a break: the right kind of company and situation.

The temporary service had placed me at some good candidates: a textile distributor that just loved me and offered me a lot to stay on with them, but it was just too darn boring. A brick manufacturer also wanted me, but it was a family business, and I would have to wait until some of the family died off just to move up, so that wouldn't work either. But a good break came in less than a year.

The heating, ventilating, and air-conditioning distribution business turned out to be it. When I hit their dock door that very first day to help with the warehousing problem for a couple of weeks, I knew I had struck gold. Here it was.

These guys had tons of business, a very good product in Rheem air-conditioning, and a very fast growing Texas economy. This had every possibility of being just what this boy had hoped for: a real opportunity. The icing on the cake was that they were disorganized in every phase of warehousing and stock checking due to growing pains and desperate for help that just wouldn't die drinking on the job or stealing from them.

That left me an opening I walked right into.

They had just hired a man by the name of Ron to run the warehouse, but I would eventually learn that he had a substance abuse problem, like the delivery driver. Never mind about that. I would cover for them, no problem. After over a year of working night and day, including very physical work for hours at a time, this was a piece of cake.

Ron didn't work much past noon, but I quickly learned what needed to be done, so I just took over, especially in the afternoons until we got the place "workable." In three days, the company offered me permanent full- or part-time work, including paying all tuition as long as I was able to bring in a C average or better in school. Johnny would actually be my direct boss and hired me. He was a combination general manager and purchasing agent, but I would work for both Ron in the warehouse and the most senior employee, John, in inside sales, wherever I was needed, including what we called "hot shot" deliveries of equipment and supplies to dealers late in the day in the smaller truck that did not require a commercial license.

They agreed to work around any school schedule I had and allowed me a key for the warehouse area to come unload semi trucks over the weekends and nights.

For both of us, that was the break of a lifetime.

Don't give a workaholic, overenergized, puzzle loving kid a key to a messed up warehouse—unless you want a change.

I was messing around with my school graph paper (remember this was 1979), and with the three trucks they had already awaiting unloading, the new inventory was not going to fit the way the place was laid out. It was going to begin to look again like that put-it-everywhere-without-organization look I was hired in to help fix the first time.

The whole problem, due to sizing of the equipment, was that the warehouse was simply laid out wrong and had been for a long time. It had just started to get noticed and become a problem because the business was growing, and pretty fast too. Along with that, the size of the inventory had to increase in tandem. We were going to have to make some changes, or this was forever going to be a problem.

Johnny came out late on Friday, a day I always worked late because we had our own gas pumps. I had become John's pet. John actually ran the company, was the most senior employee, and had forgotten more about the business than I would ever learn. But for some reason, we just loved each other like old friends from day one.

I would stay late on Fridays because it was payday, and John would let me fill up my car on the company pump after everybody left. In return, I would handle a few things when Ron or the delivery driver needed some time off in the back of the warehouse. No problem. I would have done it for free, but John knew I was constantly broke, and even though gasoline was still relatively cheap in 1979, I sure could use the free gas.

I was actually just brainstorming on the graph paper, mostly just waiting for Johnny to leave so I could get my car gassed up, when he came through the warehouse to say good-bye to me and check to make sure I could handle all the work by myself. It had been a tough day and a tough week, and three more trucks were backed up waiting for me to unload them that weekend.

Johnny saw the graph paper and said, "What is that? Our warehouse?" I said yes.

He looked at it for a good ten minutes and then said, "Do you think this will work?" I told him I was pretty sure of it, but one thing was absolutely for sure: we were going to have to try something pretty bold or get a new building. There was no third option.

He told me to go for it, work as much as I could on it that weekend. I told him I could reorganize and unload but not finish by Monday. He said he didn't care. He agreed we had to make a change and to just do what I could.

Enough said, and I almost finished. The trucks were unloaded and already gone when John, Johnny, Ron, and the president of the company, a man named Joe, pulled in for work on Monday morning.

As they walked in, I was already at work, putting on the finishing touches.

They all walked around the entire forty thousand square feet of warehouse while I was working the forklift like a madman trying to finish off. They never said a word to me, any of them. Then they were gone. About fifteen minutes later, John came out to the warehouse and signaled to me with that crooked grin of his and a curling finger to come in to the offices. The forklift was very loud inside the warehouse; we all had to signal when somebody was on it.

John sent me to Johnny's office, and he told me, "Let's go." We were on our way to the president's office. Ron was already inside, still looking kind of amazed.

Joe asked me if I would train for inside sales. They had a lot of openings coming up, and they would work out whatever I needed for school time. They would also pay for all books as well now, just for keeping a C average (what a joke). It literally meant a doubling of pay as well as full benefits, just like a full-time worker, including vacation and insurance.

That was pretty good.

A few conditions: I was to continue to help Ron in the warehouse when he needed it and still do the hot shots. I knew the customers a bit now and was occasionally asked for specifically. The rest of the time I was to work the sales counter inside, and John was going to teach me the business of heating, ventilating, and air-conditioning distribution.

I had been employed there, part time, for less than three months.

It meant I had jumped right over Ron, careerwise, as well as the other four warehouse managers in the Dallas area. A warehouse manager would usually get this opportunity first, not his helper, especially a part-time college kid. But Ron was always great about it, and we never had a problem over it.

The only thought I had in mind after that meeting, and I remember this perfectly well, was that I would be running this company in five years.

It took a little more than six, but it was a much larger company by then, and there had been many more bodies to jump over. But the president of the company when I began my career there in 1979 would wind up working for *me* by January 1986.

The first glass of lemonade had been made with the problem lemons of my life.

⬤　⬤

Training with John on the sales desk of an HVAC distributor was like going to college in the business itself. John had worked in this industry for over fifty years and was the type of person who was not only always glad to help somebody but to teach as well.

He knew he had an interested student, and he helped me in more ways than you could imagine. He began by training me on the electrical part of heating and air-conditioning, where the demand for expertise in the industry was its highest. Then he trained me on the refrigeration components, the air delivery part of the business, and on and on.

Another guardian angel.

After about three months, he began to arrange part-time, paid work for me to work with our customers who were the dealers who installed and fixed the heating and air-conditioning systems in homes and offices. This was totally invaluable experience and one that helped me throughout my career there. After a month or so of this experience, I could speak the language of an experienced HVAC contractor, as well as sell to him.

In the evenings I would stay up hours late, after whatever college assignment I had was complete, and study the manufacturers' catalogs and parts lists.

Why not? I never got tired anyway.

By now in my life, I couldn't possibly sleep past 6 a.m. and rarely went to bed before 2 a.m. A little sickness in the morning almost each day was calmed by a Sprite. The oversweating seemed to have slowed just a little, as well as the anxiety, but the learning and working energy was hitting new highs. At least I was using them.

The only difference now was that I was consciously using it for my own personal gain.

It would take me twenty-six years to admit that to myself... because this is self-abuse.

In my experience with thyroid disease, there's been an ebb and flow to the symptoms as my life went on, tidal in nature, with the tides always coming in a bit higher on me than their previous highest tide. I understand this is very similar to other people's experiences who suffer from clinical anxiety, severe hormonal problems, autoimmune diseases, and/or metabolic disease. The unfortunate, and possibly deadly, issue is that your troublesome symptoms almost always will continue to trend up in your life, each rising flow getting higher and more disruptive to either yourself or both you and someone you love who suffers this disease you both live with.

I think being focused on learning, which I loved to do, combined with an almost relentless work schedule, actually helped me "chill down" a bit for several months during my training with John. Some weekends I could sleep, some weekends not, but that was definitely better than before. I was losing the sometimes nighttime cold sweats I would experience about the dive accident. I wasn't too anxious about the future either. In Texas, you can always count on air-conditioning work, and I was making decent money at a place that cared for me and I knew I would advance with.

I was absolutely convinced nothing was wrong with me! But, of course, I was lying.

The main thing I was worried about then was not related to any of my problems anymore. I wished I had a woman in my life. I was lonely. Since I lost Wendy, my entire dating style had pretty much been like being a puppy in a puppy store, hoping a beautiful lady would come pick me up. Then I could burrow my way into her heart.

Not exactly the best way to really get out there and meet somebody special. In fact, it's pretty pathetic.

My soul mate was just around the corner of my life, but we would meet under some surprising and adversarial conditions, to say the least.

But I guess that's exactly what you'd expect out of someone like me.

●  ●

The early 1980s were a great time for growth throughout Dallas and its suburbs. We had a fantastic location
in the fastest growing suburb of Dallas in Richardson, Texas.
It just wasn't doing as well in sales as many in the company
thought it should be.

Our company was taken over before any changes were made
though. A much larger distribution group based in Houston
had bought out the six locations of our company, and that gave
them control of about 90 percent of the population of the state
of Texas.

The previous president, Joe, parachuted out completely. He
was replaced by what would become a wonderful mentor and
friend to me, Wayne.

Wayne was a type-A driver personality, due to nothing
other than a love to compete and win. He had worked for our
primary product manufacturer for several years and had risen
quite highly there before taking the opportunity with what is a
very important area to an air-conditioning manufacturing company: Texas. Keep in mind that maybe 15 to 20 percent of our
primary manufacturer's gross sales would come from one distributor now, so it was very important to them *who* was running
the place. It made a difference to their entire company. They
didn't want to make a living out of training executives for their
distributors, but in this case, it was tolerated very well because
of its overall strategic importance.

Wayne wound up living less than five minutes from our
Richardson store, and after his first visit to that store, he later
told me in confidence he wanted a change.

It never took Wayne long to make a decision. On anything.

When he called me into his office after he had been there
about two weeks, he asked me if I had time to go have a beer
after closing, but not at the local place just up the road where

all the employees regularly met after work, but a different, professional-type bar.

Of course I could and was happy to. This had to be pretty important.

I was a little worried he might be changing the school reimbursement plan, but I didn't get the feeling he was thinking about that at all. Besides, I thought he would have told me that kind of thing right there in his office; it's just business. As it turned out, he would support me more than anybody in the company on virtually every single issue of my career while he was there, including education.

What I learned later on in my career there was when Wayne wanted to get you alone, you were toast.

Whenever there was a really tough, lousy job or assignment, you would get taken to a nice bar or go with him to the Texas Rangers using the company season tickets, or a super restaurant of some note. Wherever Wayne could get you one-on-one was his tactic. He was very, very persuasive, especially when he had you to himself. He never lost to me at one of those matches, I have to admit. He got me to do it every single time … and some crummy assignments too.

But he couldn't have possibly talked me *out* of the new position he wanted me to take: the management of the Richardson store. He was ready to trust one of the most important growth stores in the entire company, a highly visible flagship operation, to a twenty-two-year-old kid who had worked there about eleven months and whom he had known about two weeks.

Of course, he admitted there could be a few problems, like the dozen other counter salesmen in our other branches who had been dying for that job since the store opened and my jumping right over them, and the problems at the sales branch itself (which were much worse than either of us could have imagined). The assistant manager there named Randy, whose attitude had begun to slip lately, would also be insulted as I jumped over him as well. And maybe a few other things as well. He wasn't sure just how bad things were to be honest with me.

Sounded just like old home week to me. And I really didn't have any questions.

Just like with Coach K, I knew what he wanted. Why waste time talking about it? The whole deal was finished in one beer. We went ahead and had a second beer, just for fun really. He and I had both gotten what we wanted. He got his man in charge of the flagship operation. I got the most desirable promotion available. We both won that time.

I didn't work an exact salary figure out. I just told him that I trusted him to make that right if he trusted me with this position, and, of course, he did. It's a great tactic to use with proud men like Wayne. You would almost always get more if you made them do it than if you tried to negotiate your own. Try this; it works with the right kind of up-front supervisor who has risen up the ladder some on his or her own. I doubt it works with the cheapskate type of boss. I have been lucky enough to not have had many of those.

We closed as we left the bar with what day he wanted me to start. The next day was a Friday and a pay period, so he would make the change himself tomorrow and close out the cash portion of the branch. I would take over Monday. The much longer commute got me an extra bonus, unlimited (read that, personal) use of the company pickup, including fuel. This also gave us the power to run "hot shot" deliveries out of a branch operation, a new and untried option, which we learned to use very effectively and quite profitably to the point of outright envy and anger about fairness from the other branch managers.

I said nothing the next day about what had happened to anybody but John, who already knew anyway, and he wasn't telling. John was probably the biggest reason I got this break to begin with. It all happened so fast there was little time for a lot of complaining from those I'd jumped. But frankly, I wouldn't have cared if there was, and now I had very important allies, as well as myself, to help "stomp on it" if backlash occurred to ruffle the feathers of the most recent resurfacing problems of my disease: my regrowing ego.

That type of attitude both was and is wrong in so many ways, but it's business, and I tend to try to separate the two a bit when it comes to personal ambition. More importantly to many of us—and those who love us—is that this type of attitude and behavior also contributes to substantially worsening your anxiety and increasing your self-abuse and denial.

It doesn't matter if you want to realize or accept it. It will happen to you anyway. At least it does in my experience and in the experiences of others too. You can run but not hide from disease.

And you'll probably continue to get worse, not better. Just like I did.

*But this was okay,* I justified quickly in my mind. *Wasn't taking these "lemons" and using them for money and power the master plan anyway? And what had just occurred was sure more money and power than ever before in my life, by a long shot. Isn't that enough evidence for everyone to see?*

*Let me just keep repeating this as fast as I can. This has got to be the answer to ending this anxiousness and finding happiness. It has to be.*

•   •

Walking in to the Richardson branch early on that Monday was just about like walking into a smelly public toilet. You couldn't wait to get out. I wouldn't have wanted to do any business there. I was surprised we had any customers at all for that store.

The place reeked of cigar smoke from the previous manager. The floors, walls, drop ceiling, warehouse, bathrooms, and office were filthy. There's just no other way to put it. It was a complete mess from top to bottom, inside and out.

I got kind of mad just looking around the place. I would have been absolutely livid if I had been the owner.

I hadn't begun to check the audit of sale orders or tickets yet. That would have to wait; everybody was sure there had been inventory shrink anyway, so that wouldn't be news. First, this place had to be remade into a professional distribution operation from a pigsty. And that was not going to be a one-week job.

But a situation like that can be the opportunity of your life. I tried very hard to make it so.

I was going to need some help, in the form of money, to recover the operation. Wayne was more than generous—no budget, just keep it as low as you can. I told him we had to repaint, recarpet, and refloor quite a bit, but he did not waiver. With Wayne, that meant get to it; it was due yesterday.

So I went to work cleaning up, and then Randy showed up for work a few minutes late.

I introduced myself as Clay, the new manager, and it went over like a lead balloon.

I never held Randy accountable for the problems we had at first with work ethic and customer service. He had never been properly trained and felt underutilized mostly due to a complete lack of leadership from his previous manager. Randy was not only very intelligent with a very quick wit, but he could, and did, become one very successful salesman. He honestly had been given no chance working in the situation he was in.

But it didn't take long for us to build up to an incident—about four days to be exact.

It occurred on the Friday following the Monday I took over. He was still a bit mad at being jumped over, and my work pace demands bordered upon the fanatic. It put him in a tough spot, but it was going to have to be my way or the highway. I knew you had to run your business, or it will run you.

The cleaning and painting of the sales area, offices, and bathrooms was difficult, dirty, and filthy work. I knew that, but we were working side by side on everything. I have never, and still make it a policy to this day, to not ask someone to do something I would not do or have not already done myself.

So I told him, "Come on and pick it up, man. We gotta get with this. There's a bunch to do." And that started it.

He told me I could take it and put it someplace, and I said, "Hit the door, and don't let it bust your butt on the way out." He cooled it right there, and so did I.

I gave it a half-minute truce because I was afraid of losing it. I was glad I did that too.

He told me he didn't want to quit or get fired, but he hadn't had a chance to become the manager there and had worked for the company longer than I had, plus had the biggest jerk in the company to work for. I said I understood—I really did—that I had John to train me and suggest me for this job, an opportunity he had never had. I also said that a manager that kept porno books in the men's bathroom at work was not the type of guy to be working around, and that that had sucked for sure. That much alone had killed his chances to be promoted, especially with an executive like Wayne.

The only thing I could promise him was that if he would just work with me, he would indeed be the next manager at that branch. I could just about guarantee it. But things had to change, starting with his attitude. When you become a manager with financial responsibility and staff, or want to become one, especially at this young stage of your career, you are going to have to make a decision to become a "company man," or the company has made a mistake in trusting you. I absolutely would not be that mistake under any circumstances, nor let him be one either. He would be gone first. Period.

Turns out we talked until almost 6:30 p.m., when we normally closed at 5 p.m., and on a Friday to boot. Randy had a lot of important things to say and very good ideas we could try. He just needed somebody to listen to him. He knew the customers pretty well, what they liked and didn't like, as well as what many of the root problems of the branch really were. I made several notes on a yellow note pad, not just as a sign of respect but because I knew I was actually hearing the truth that would help us both.

We took that note pad the following Monday and made it into the to-do list.

We also talked about our ambitions for the future, that there definitely was a future with this company, and how we could get there. Somebody who had ambition like Randy had could definitely be saved as a worker, and maybe become a friend to me as well.

We did become friends, ultimately very good friends, as well as teammates that day. It was a turning-point time for everybody, including our company. Few knew it though.

That was the first day that would mark the flagship branch really becoming a flagship. It was also a time that marked when two of the most important future managers of that company were "corporately born."

Too bad my disease would soon grow to the point that I would soon be physically and mentally unable to routinely give problems that same half-minute truce I had done so successfully with Randy. It would cost me dearly over the next thirty years, in every facet of my life.

●　●

The to-do list had been nearly completed in about two months. Both customers and company staff alike had been shocked by the changes. We still weren't totally finished in the warehouse, but the office and sales area were one of the best looking in the company now.

The only person who hadn't seen it, and lived less than five minutes away, was Wayne.

He called me one rainy morning, about 8:30 a.m. to ask if he could come by. It was a great sign of respect he continued to show for me during both of my operational manager duties over the next few years. He would never call another manager before he came by their branches. He didn't and shouldn't have to. He was the second most senior executive of the company and a fractional owner. But the showing of that respect meant a great deal to me, and to give the man credit, he always knew what button of mine to push.

I told him it was about time he got his butt over; we were getting worn out waiting.

He tried to hide his shock when he came in, but it showed anyway. I saw it from the back where I was stuck in my office. Randy took him on a grand tour over the whole place—inside and out—just like he had never seen the operation. I was totally focused right then on closing a brand new customer we had stolen away from a competitor brand just the previous week who called me to sign up as a new dealer right after I hung up with Wayne. Over seven thousand dollars of commercial rooftop units got ordered before I let that customer get out of my office that morning, with a check and a completed credit account application to go with it. Wayne would have to wait. I was sorry. I knew he had called and everything, but this was serious business, and Wayne understood serious business came first. So he just went ahead and toured around the facility a second time, chatted with Randy a good bit, wasting a solid forty-five minutes or so.

Finally I closed the customer and got free. This one customer alone would become a fifty-thousand-dollar-a-year account we had never even been able to sell a thermostat to before. Wayne knew of the customer's importance, and, of course, Randy reminded him of it as well. Probably a couple of times I bet.

Wayne stayed for about five to ten minutes with me in my office when I got free, never even taking his raincoat off. We just chatted a minute; then he left. He never said a single word to me about the changes or anything we were doing. I honestly think he was a little overwhelmed, and that was a tough thing to do to Wayne, believe me.

He never returned to the branch again while I was manager. Not a single time.

This was one of the easiest periods of my life. Able to work with little supervision and nearly complete autonomy removed a great deal of anxiety from my life, as it would from anyone's. It allowed a growing and blossoming professionally during this period that is unmatched in my opinion to this day. Perhaps this is because this would turn out to be the lowest point of my anxiety and physical symptoms I would experience for more than twenty-eight years.

·  ·

There was one tiny little problem left at the very end of the branch renovation: parts. Or rather, the pile-of-trash parts that were in stock that nobody would buy because they were worthless.

Parts are a very important piece of the HVAC distribution business. Not only do your contractors count on you to keep good parts inventory for their warranty work, but they need one-stop-type shopping experiences where they can get all they need for a day or two's work at one supply house. With the parts we had, we simply could not supply that, even though we were beginning to be a strong force with our equipment sales.

The other tiny part of that problem was that our acquiring company had paid for those junk parts and thought they were usable and salable inventory. Sorry folks, they're not.

And you can bet that caused a nasty stink all around going back to the previous ownership. But I was out of that part of it; it was a corporate matter. Just don't kill the messenger please. I still needed some parts to sell and help with warranty.

Wayne argued with me for a couple of days but then relented; he had to. My parts sales were fractionally low to our equipment business, so it wasn't a staff problem. It was an inventory problem that needed a solution. The other branches weren't stocked with either enough or the exact style of parts we needed at that location for a transfer to help much.

So I had an order pad now, and when Johnny approved, I could stock my own branch.

Looks like I hadn't spent all those hours on nights when I couldn't sleep with the parts catalogs for nothing after all.

My mentor, John, in the main office had always ordered Honeywell boxed parts for the sale parts to dealers and Rheem plain-boxed parts of Honeywell product for warranty use, as required by our manufacturer. I had noticed one important point about that.

We could buy the exact replacement parts that worked on about five other manufacturers' units plus our own: the exact Honeywell part, only from Rheem and for a substantial discount due to our volume and the plain packaging.

A very substantial discount.

So that was exactly what I began to do. Our branch margins and parts sales exploded almost overnight. In less than six months after taking over, the Richardson branch officially became the number one branch in the entire twelve-branch company in growth and profitability.

From worst to first—literally.

Unfortunately, the Honeywell representative exploded too when she found out her bread and butter parts sales to us were down a good bit "due to that new Richardson manager," Johnny would tell her. Seems like a couple of our other branch managers were learning some new tricks too! Normally I could have cared less, even laughed and been quite proud about cracking a rep and their program like I had done.

Except this time. Turns out the Honeywell rep was a wonderfully friendly, charming, poised, and beautiful, long-legged lady—that I fell smooth in love with. Her name was Abby.

But she was pretty mad at me right then over what I was doing. I couldn't and didn't blame her one bit for it either.

Talk about career problems! And just when things had been going so well too.

•  •

It was a great time in my life working at the branch after Randy and I had cleared the air and put the place in order. We were in the sweet spot of growth in the country. This time period of almost a year of relaxed teamwork, high productivity, with positive focus and leadership, definitely marked a low ebb in all my symptoms.

Many of the most nagging symptoms had already eased up on me substantially. My skin, especially from the knee down, began to improve and look much healthier. Morning nausea had almost completely ceased, but I still wouldn't eat until late in the day, "Just in case," I told myself. I began to regrow light hair on my back, legs, and upper arms that had disappeared after the stress of the dive accident. I could control my temperature much better, and I had little moodiness nor cause for much anxiety.

Except that I had fallen in love, and that meant decision time.

Abby offered me what somebody with anxiety issues or hyperthyroidism desperately needed. Pure love and calm in a storm of anxiousness. The ability to see through and forgive the occasional unexplained anger. Devotion to the hopes and dreams of a better future not only for herself but for those around her.

I decided this time there would be no lying if we stuck it. I would duck the issues with her whenever I could, skirt around them with minimum truths shaded in a positive way. Plus, by now, I had an arsenal of excuses, jokes, and subject diversions that nobody, even doctors and very smart bosses, could fight their way through.

Privately I tried, with less and less success as time went by, to hide and deny the not-so-visible symptoms—growing anxiety that had no cause, confusing me more than usual, as this was a happy time. But love can breed some natural anxiety on its own.

I was experiencing occasional depression, also misunderstood, but not without reason. However, it did seem to be a bit worse than I could remember from past bouts. Little wonder. It's a natural offshoot of being sick for a long time. Clinical depression can occur for this reason whether the sufferer is diagnosed and understands their medical condition or not.

Overall though, I was feeling better, and my anxiety level was way down. Being with Abby just seemed natural and right.

But there had to be no lying. I couldn't lose this one. She might be it.

I hoped that maybe over time I could talk these things through with somebody really special like Abby was. I was constantly thinking about her even though we had only met a few days before.

That's how it's always been for me. I'll wait forever (just like that puppy in the store) for the right woman if need be, but when the right one comes along, I'm going to burrow in, and it's going to take dynamite to blast me out. And I'll do it quick too.

So I got ready to burrow in.

Abby and I initially tried to keep any relationship a secret due to the many conflicts of interest that were possible between a buyer and a vendor. But once it started, we let it officially out. Of course, we had fooled *exactly no one*. You never do.

We went out six times in the first seven days after our first date.

Less than a month after our first date, I moved into an apartment complex next door to Abby's complex so we could be together constantly. My place was less than three hundred yards away from her front door.

After less than three months, we began to discuss a lifetime future together.

# Climbing the Ladders of Symptoms and Success

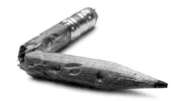

Late in November, not one full year into my management of the branch, I got a call late morning from Wayne. He wanted Joe, the new sales manager, and me to meet him for drinks at a bar about halfway between my branch and the main offices that afternoon and asked if I could I make it. Sure I could. I had school that afternoon but would skip for this (I wouldn't dare tell Wayne that), but I was losing total interest in college since becoming a manager and was barely making Bs in simple classes. I was only getting those Bs mostly due to my charming of the teaching assistants. This is a crazy aspect of anxiety-based lack of confidence that I experienced all the time. You can charm the pants right off anybody you don't have a vested interest in, but if it really counts to you personally, you'll run away a lot due to fear and lack of confidence.

It also hadn't escaped my notice that I was now older than a lot of the other students.

*Let's go have a beer and see what's on Wayne's mind,* I thought.

It was another tough assignment, the worst sales territory

in the Dallas/Fort Worth region. The most underserviced with representation for several years. The slowest growing of the Dallas suburbs and tons of small towns spread out all over from Waco to east Texas.

I didn't want this job and began to argue and argue hard. "I have only been at Richardson less than a year. I'm jumping again over a bunch of branch managers who want territories; give them this one! I haven't got a good enough car for an outside sales job. I still need the company truck!" On and on I went. I was sure I would get a chance sooner or later in the Richardson territory if I could hold out, and that was almost becoming a retirement job the way Randy and I had things going.

I lost out. Wayne won again. He always did.

The new sales manager, Joe, whom we had for what had now become the northern division of our fast growing company, was also stolen from the Rheem executive group. He was not one bit easier than Wayne on me, then or in the future, and really had a rugged persuasive streak that had carried him up tougher ladders than I would ever be.

But make no mistake, this wasn't any Richardson branch slam dunk of nearly guaranteed success. This was the worst territory you could get in the whole company. You can also read that as the worst opportunity they had to offer in a promotion.

But of course, give it some credit; it was a promotion at least and had a chance, however slim, of making some commission money as well.

What they never told me was that territory was a lot more important than virtually anybody else in the company knew. The ultimatum from one of our manufacturers was that if I wasn't successful in selling a very high-end line of equipment in and around the Waco area of my territory, the company was going to lose the line. The whole equipment and parts line, and in every branch of the company.

It was probably best I didn't know that in retrospect. That's real pressure, and I could have pressed too hard and blown it with the kind of problems I had.

Wayne solved the car problem temporarily; he sold me his own Buick, cheap.

Plus, I gained a friend to this day in Joe, a man who really taught me the art of salesmanship, as well as many important and necessary aspects of professional sales management. The skills and tactics he taught me I use every day to this day. Another guardian angel.

It wasn't a total loss, but boy, I sure wanted a chance at anything other than this area. You see, that sales territory also included the area of Dallas that I grew up in.

●  ●

My financial position had changed dramatically in the last year and a half, and I received my first bonus check for the management of the Richardson branch. Three thousand dollars! The biggest bonus ever given to date to a branch manager.

I checked with my roommate, Tom, whose brother was a stockbroker and supposedly a really good one. Tom and I agreed to buy some stock. He had saved some money too, but we had done no research. It was the 1980s stock market lows, and as I have always done and advocated, "Buy 'em when they're on sale." So we would. Tom's brother had a great idea company called *National Patent Development* that looked really good to him in the next year or so.

Sounded good to me. I looked it up in an S&P book I had him send me, and sure enough this stock had been put on sale, about 35 percent or so, and there looked to be some future prospects. I bought all I had with that bonus in NPD at around eight dollars a share. I sold it late the next year, for about thirty bucks a share, and I was hooked forever.

I had always loved the markets and had actually traded stocks with my dad when I was nine years old at the old Merrill, Lynch, Pierce, Fenner, and Smith office in downtown Dallas. I never made or lost much money. I could only trade a few shares, but I just loved the whole atmosphere. Had I ever gotten a college degree, I believe I would have tried to go into investment banking.

I didn't know that within just a few years I would wind up owning a small brokerage.

But I was addicted in 1981 to the market. It has never let me go to this day.

But lately I noticed I had begun to attract my old adversary again: anxiety. The morning nausea had returned again, at this point in time causing me to be unable to eat anything until very late in the day (you could also read that "until the workday was over"). My skin had begun to develop red sores of dryness that would occasionally bleed a little, and I had begun to have dandruff that I was unable to control with over-the-counter dandruff shampoos.

I was managing to hide most of the recurring symptoms pretty well, but I felt I was going to have to deal with these problems pretty soon, just not right now. I simply didn't have the time. I had just gotten this new promotion and had a very tough job ahead. I needed a new car and some better clothes. As soon as I got this work stuff under control, I'd take care of it. *Take it to the bank!* I thought.

Sound familiar?

But it would be almost thirty years before I "took care of it," or rather, it nearly took care of me.

● ●

Even though we were still mired in the 1981–1982 recession, I managed to grow the territory 35 percent that next year. It was not tops in the company by far; that honor went to a lovely lady and wonderful friend who had the Richardson territory.

Sometimes being a company man means taking the assignments you know you can't win with. Wayne and Joe knew that. They had had to do it themselves before. They also knew I had taken the heat off of the sales pressure from the equipment manufacturer about our sales in Waco. So I was rewarded pretty well with a luxury weeklong trip to Acapulco at the Las Brisas hotel, and believe it or not, 35 percent commissions.

Abby and I had a fabulous time in Mexico, but I contracted the usual tourist disease and returned home to promptly lose thirty-five pounds in three weeks.

In retrospect, the stress of the turista had exploded my disease now into huge weight swings I would suffer until my true diagnosis. Things were definitely getting worse, but they couldn't have diagnosed me accurately then anyway. The sonogram and the blood-thyroid testing equipment had not been invented yet.

But that didn't keep the symptoms from coming back stronger than ever. I was really stressed out about how I looked, and so were my coworkers. I was forced to wear workout shorts, sweatpants, and undershirts under my clothes to help fill them out because I had no budget to immediately buy a whole new wardrobe. It happened too fast.

I originally thought the perspiration that began to occur was due to all the clothing I was wearing in layers, but that wasn't it. The temperature control issue of my long undiagnosed thyroid disease had begun to rear its ugly head with the sweating again. Except now I also had an occasional freezing problem again as well—without warning at times, sweating at the head, hands, and underarms with freezing cold feet.

I knew something was wrong. *I must still have the turista!* I thought. I went back to the doctors for additional testing, and it was negative, except for a small leukocyte (infection-fighting white blood cells) count the doctors thought I had developed due to a renewed but dormant symptom of allergies.

Allergies! Where the heck did that come back from? Allergies can come and go? I hadn't had those symptoms since a few months after the dive accident, and then they slowly went away on their own. But the doctors countered that allergies could come and go, especially if you change climate zones or as we age.

Not again, no way! These guys must be crazy.

Turns out they *were* crazy. I shouldn't have listened. But misdiagnosis is very common and routine with thyroid disease sufferers. I relented to their arguments and began allergy shots along with oral medication, which would needlessly continue for twenty years. Also lasting for the next twenty years was a growing frustration and mistrust of the medical community that many of us with thyroid disease, whether diagnosed or not, share.

Desperate to strike out in every direction for any help, I began to try herbal medications, Chinese medicine, and eventually holistic healers to help the ever-growing sinus problem that would ebb and flow higher and higher despite routine use of all prescribed medications. But of course, those options didn't (and couldn't) help me either.

I slowly began to regain the lost weight and hold food down better over the next six months, and thankfully I had Abby to help and support me. I don't know where I'd be right now if she had not been there for me so many times over the last twenty-six years.

There's no question that the turista episode definitely marked a turning point in the ebb of symptoms I had been enjoying for almost two years. I was definitely depressed now, both by how I looked (this has caused me to develop a clothes horse phobia once I gained some measure of financial success, a condition that continues to this day) as well as how I felt. I was constantly sick to my stomach, and not just in the mornings but almost all day a lot. I had lost the hair off my back and legs again. The worst part by far was more moodiness than I had known in years; all these symptoms had begun again in earnest.

The next flows I would experience would be much higher than ever and include many additional health and behavior problems it would take me years to overcome.

•  •

The territory was growing slightly, but late in the spring, we lost Joe back to Rheem, and I lost a real guardian angel. It was a big loss for me, personally and professionally.

The following year of 1982 was much more difficult for me. The new sales manager and I simply did not get along. He had been a sales rep for many years and had moved down from Missouri to sell heavy commercial product and had been given the promotion to sales manager. Certainly I was not jealous of his promotion, not wanting the job at all. That had nothing to do with our inability to work together; it was strictly business. Or, more specifically, lack of the type of professional sales support and leadership all of the outside sales staff had grown to expect. Things were not working out with many other reps as well.

The anxiety and stress from the combination of disease, a comparatively tough sales territory, and poor professional leadership had risen to a new level, causing me to question both my job as well as my sanity. I feared I could be suffering from mental illness like I believed my mom had. I was becoming terrified about that possibility. It was taking a lot out of me just to act like nothing was wrong.

I began to visit with a multitude of medical specialists. Internists, neurologists, general practitioners, and orthopedic doctors. There were as many opinions as specialties to my variety of symptoms.

Unfortunately, none were right; the medical community still had no definitive test to run on me for a positive and final diagnosis. That was still twenty years away.

Commission sales is a terrific anxiety builder on its own, but in my case, I got the side benefit of being able to use my ability to "act", highly developed from years of denial, to its fullest. This can be a big help to a sales career but is in reality self-abuse. I felt I was balancing the increased professional demands with the growing anxiety pretty well, but you can't manage a diseased gland without medical treatment no matter how hard you try. Irritability began to return as it always did, and now I would find it so out of control I would occasionally fly off in anger at anyone around me, including people I didn't know, for very little reason.

To try to counter this behavior that was not only confusing but unwanted, I began to research self-help books on relaxation and anger management techniques. I had no luck with any of them, and this only increased the frustration and anxiety. The vicious circles of symptoms not only continued but grew in intensity, regardless of how hard I tried and what I would do to stop them.

I began to look around at other job opportunities. I think Wayne could tell or knew. I was about to quit my third straight very good job because I believed the jobs were making me sick. As perplexing as that might appear, keep in mind that several recent visits to doctors about my myriad of symptoms had given me nothing but misdiagnosis frustration beyond belief. All I was doing was simply reverting to being alone as a solution again. I didn't know what else to do.

Early summer, I was in the offices after closing a very large new account, and Wayne called me in his office unexpectedly. He chatted around some, and then he asked me what was wrong.

I told him, straight out, we weren't getting the sales support we needed and that was really his responsibility and he was fumbling the ball big time. Looking back on it, I'm glad we had the kind of relationship we had, or I could have gotten thrown out on my behind for talking like that to a senior executive. But the sales management we had then was actually starting to cost me money in lost orders—big orders too. The combination of a poor sales territory and bad sales management had me at the end of my rope. So as they say, I told him the nasty truth because I figured I was looking for a job when I found this one, and I was more than fed up with it by this time.

It knocked Wayne back in his chair. He simply asked me if I had anything else.

I said, "No, but you asked, and I have never lied to you about business, ever."

That sales manager was gone the next Friday.

In irony, my fiancée was laid off by Honeywell that same Friday in June 1982, due strictly to "lack of seniority." This despite a more than stellar overall sales performance that included about 50-percent sales growth with our company alone. Talk about poor timing; we had just begun to discuss wedding dates for a few months in the future, perhaps November, when that bombshell hit.

And a new behavior problem began, one that I would fight for almost thirty years.

Hate. Long-lasting, deep, revenge-oriented hate. A hate that could burn for years.

I took names of the Honeywell managers involved in her being laid off when she was the number two rep out of ten reps in that group. I wouldn't forget those names, at least until I had busted them down or out of Honeywell and our industry.

It was less than forty-eight hours after Abby was laid off until Wayne called. He wanted to go to the Texas Rangers baseball game the next Thursday night and wanted to know if I could come.

When have I ever refused? Of course.

It wasn't the sales manager's job. I knew that. He already had a man lined up for that in advance. It had just been our very frank discussion that had broken the camel's back on the previous manager. It would never possibly work for a twenty-three-year-old, two-and-a-half-year employee to supervise more than forty salespeople, the vast majority of which were more than twice his age and had spent their entire professional lives in the industry. Besides, I wouldn't have taken it, even for Wayne. I just thought I was finally going to get a better territory.

But it was worse, much worse: Oklahoma City.

"Oh, and don't Abby's folks live there and have a business there too?" he asked.

Of course, he already knew the answer. He rarely asked a question like that he didn't know the answer to before you opened your mouth.

I mean, you had to give Wayne credit. He could and would punch every button you had.

But oh no. Never! Move to Oklahoma City from Dallas? Are you crazy? A University-of-Texas-at-Dallas boy move to the heart of Oklahoma Sooner country? Replace a manager that has a substance-abuse problem? A completely different type and style of equipment and supply market that I had completely no experience in? No, absolutely not. It's just simply impossible.

I moved up about two weeks later. Abby would follow at the end of the month.

We rearranged our wedding plans for the following November of 1983. A year delay.

But the hate hadn't stopped burning. I had only hidden it away for a few days. I knew this new position would put me in a position of power with vendors that few enjoyed. I planned to make use of my hate for a negative result for many others. Self-abuse at its finest.

Anger had always been a part of my life, ready to rise with any excuse, primarily due to disease, but this episode of feelings was beyond anger. Abby had been hurt by the layoff, and that provided plenty of excuse for me. I began an attack on those managers at Honeywell involved in what I believed was an unfair firing. Beginning first by buying from other vendors, then refusing to work with the managers involved in her termination decision, and finally, threatening to move what business left we were doing with them to a competitor, ending all relationship with them entirely.

It did have some side benefit. They found room immediately for her at the Oklahoma City branch as soon as we moved there, only in a slightly different division. Amazing luck I guess.

It took me four years, but I got it done. By the time I stopped crushing those I felt responsible, they were little more than floor workers in the controls division assembly line.

Not much of a lifetime achievement to discuss in front of many. It's resulted in an episode I'm not proud of in review, like a lot of other episodes you've read about by now in this book (as well as some to come unfortunately). In fact, I'm ashamed of what I did then. I bring it up to show you another way how *not* to deal with our problems by not making the same mistakes I have made. Anger has cost me an awful lot, including some things I will never live down.

I've battled anger tooth and nail every day of my life until I was properly diagnosed. But it's different now, if only because I understand what's wrong.

If you find you can't or won't get over any serious anger issues in your life and hate has begun to develop or has already developed, please listen to me. You desperately need to see an MD right away. You very well could find that you aren't really angry at whatever issue or person you thought you were angry at. You're really angry—like I was—that something's wrong with you and you don't know what it is. In my case, I was expressing the terrible frustration with anger toward the wrong things and at the wrong people.

Sometimes you'll wind up hurting people that you love and/or that love you with misdirected anger.

If you won't go to a doctor for yourself, will you go for them and their happiness?

T he fifteen months at the Oklahoma City branch were not the highlight of my career.

When Wayne called me the first time, after about thirty days there, he asked what I thought we should do about the branch.

I said, "Sell it."

He laughed, but not so happily. He told me to stick it out. I said I would for a while.

I had managed to get every perk in the book before I went though. A brand new sedan company car, sign my own expense accounts, unlimited autonomy with staff and ordering. I had made the list so big, I was sure Wayne would tell me to go jump.

He didn't. So I was stuck. For a while at least.

Wayne called me up again right after Halloween when I had sold a huge order to the largest contractor in the state we had never done a dollar's worth of business with and asked me what I thought now. "Should we open that branch in Tulsa now?"

I said, "Sell it."

There was no laugh from him, only silence this time. I guess what people might call that awkward pause. He changed the subject to a positive one.

I never told Wayne to sell that branch so many times just because I was unhappy, or that the previous manager had left a real mess to deal with in so many ways. It was purely business. The type and style of equipment and supplies sold were very different in Oklahoma than in Texas. It was a different temperature zone with greatly different methods of construction used. It simply did not fit in with the rest of our branches.

I'd had a good deal of experience in not fitting in for the last twenty years or so. I knew it when I saw it, like many of us with thyroid disease understand this sort of issue pretty well, be it business or personal.

I had managed to replace the customers from what had

basically been good old boys who had liked the previous manager and did business with him on that basis, regardless of how poorly the operations went, to a different customer base—one that was much more professional in nature, larger in size, and had no time for poor operations or service so they would give their business to the best vendor in open competition.

That winning vendor was becoming our branch operation now more and more throughout the central Oklahoma area. The only staff change needed to make that happen was the previous manager had to be let go. The rest of that staff was fine. They just needed leadership and focus.

I became even less popular with some of our longer-term customers loyal to the previous manager after that firing happened. But I couldn't care less. I wasn't up there for a popularity contest; I was up there to make the company, and myself, *money*. But at the eleven-month mark, right before our beautiful wedding in the Blue Room of the Oklahoma Governor's Mansion, I began to reinterview in Dallas for jobs with competitors.

I knew I'd get to feeling better and be much happier back in Texas. I was sure.

I couldn't hide or choke down all my constantly redeveloping problems from my beautiful new wife very long. The most visible of these was skin problems, and when they started to occur again in response to the stress and anxiety of the move and the promotion, she said, "You are going to go to the doctor!"

I guess, at age twenty-seven in 1984, you would have to say I became a "clinical" case of thyroid disease.

That's right. About twenty-five years before I would "blow out." But I didn't know it. Nobody else did either.

The symptoms presented visually with my skin, like so many times before, also on my back this time, as well as the legs. By now, my skin had begun to crack and bleed from dryness so severe it caused round sores. Hair had disappeared once again from my upper legs, arms, and most of my back. It was immediately misdiagnosed by the dermatology specialist as a chronic dry skin problem, similar to eczema. I was given a strong hydrocortisone cream to use, which did immediately stop the cracking and bleeding. Only it gave me a kind of waxy, shiny skin area that looked nothing like the rest of my body.

That was going to have to do for now. I knew I could swear Abby to secrecy about the visible problems; they didn't appear to be related to either my anger or rarely discussed anxiety problem to either us or the doctors I had seen so far. I would have to make due with the treatment given and hide the skin problems with expensive clothing. This solution also helped feed an ego that needed to grow as the denial did.

What a terrific double benefit, I thought.

What I didn't know then, that I learned a few years later, was that in addition to my undiagnosed thyroid disease, I had developed a full-blown vitamin A deficiency I still suffer from to this day. This was despite the fact that I regularly ate red meat and had a fairly healthy diet. I had also taken general vitamin supplements for many years since athletics in school. My body simply didn't absorb vitamin A anymore due to the years of untreated thyroid disease.

It's not known scientifically why many, but not all, people with hormonal imbalances, anxiety, thyroid, metabolic, and autoimmune diseases contract vitamin-A deficiencies right alongside their main problem(s). But many times we do.

And the effects, as well as the misdiagnosis, can be fatal.

Skin problems can also continue a cycle of anxieties, fear, and depression, continuing to worsen the situation and even more viciously spin the cycle on us.

If you have constant or very chronic skin dryness and cracking—what some folks might call an "alligator" or "riverbed" look to the skin on your lower legs, back, or arms—you may have a serious medical problem that will never be healed by a cream, dietary changes, or supplements. Your skin will only get worse and worse. You must take the symptoms list from this book and go to your doctor within a few days. *You may be very sick.*

I did not tell the doctors treating my skin problems of any of my "other" problems I had. Problems like anxiety, temperature control, constantly changing weight, and unexplained irritability. By now I didn't trust doctors, and I was sure all these different symptoms weren't related. But I've learned now you're always sure when you're in denial.

But in late 1984 it was decided I was headed back to Texas. There had been big changes in the company.

That mattered little to me at that point. By then, I knew I would not be long in the company anymore. I couldn't make enough money to satisfy me that way. I had learned what the top executives were making in our industry through the interview processes.

Besides, I had a new mistress now. The stock and commodities markets had become my new nighttime courtesan. I had plenty of time and energy, and I couldn't sleep anyway.

•　•

Our company was owned by a NYSE listed firm based in New York City, but they were rarely heard from. In fact, I never met any of them until all hell broke loose when Wayne and our company president resigned in late 1984 to take the same product line I had saved for the company during my Waco territory just a few years earlier. They were to open three branches they owned entirely themselves with that brand as their feature line. In a few minutes, Wayne went from mentor and guardian angel to competitor.

I immediately received a call from the vice-chairman of our

holding company, and he asked to meet me in Dallas. I was happy to.

I also received a call from Wayne very soon after. They would not open an operation in Oklahoma, for a number of reasons, but he still wanted to work together. I thanked him for that and told him we would talk very soon about it and that I wanted to wish him the very best of luck in his new business.

I should have been more honest then and told him the truth about my leaving this industry sooner than later. Instead I said nothing of the kind. I was really just depressed about losing another trusted guardian angel of my professional life.

My meeting with the vice-chairman went very well, and he was a man to the point, just like I liked to be. He allowed me to be more than frank with him on every issue we both had and ultimately wound up doing exactly as I suggested. He also raised my pay to well above a sales manager's usual range. Over fifty thousand a year, plus expenses and luxury car as a twenty-seven-year-old with no college degree in 1984, was not a bad deal.

It just wasn't enough for me.

I told him, "Sell it," like I had told Wayne; then Abby and I would like to move to Austin and I would manage the under-performing division there.

We did sell it in about twenty-two days and at a good, fair price.

So it was set that Abby and I would move on December 29, 1984, to Austin. I would become the central division sales manager.

By God, if something like that won't make you happy, nothing would. Right?

*Right!*

• •

There was little in my time with the company in Austin that would make me happy. I think the senior executive of the division and the newly hired president of the company thought I was after their jobs.

At least, they always acted that way a lot.

The constant comments from both of them about who thought they were really the boss aimed at me on the surface in jest were really quite revealing of their own real fears and maybe closer to the truth than any of us cared to admit. A close attachment with a member of our holding company's Board of Directors I had developed earlier during the company civil war threatened them as well, I think. My attitude of lacking of much interest, respect, or in the case of superiors, fear of retribution, were other clues they thought I was trying to bust them out of their jobs. I can understand where in their eyes, a twenty-six-year-old who had jumped over hundreds around him in so few years had to have only one objective.

But they never had the courage to ask me. I guess they just assumed I had risen so far and so fast that the only ultimate resolution for me was that I run the company. But I had no intention of doing that. I was already gone in my mind. But I guess you would have to also say that I wasn't as forthcoming about many of these things as I could have been either.

By the time my senior executive figured it out, I was already well on my way out.

I'd worked around executives since I was in the internship program. I understood the incidences of anxiety, egomania, anger, and depression sometimes went hand in hand with the job. I continued to rationalize that my own problems with many of these exact same issues were just due to the routine pressure of executive leadership. I never allowed myself to face up to the fact that I had been troubled with most of these symptoms since I was five years old.

It wasn't pressure; it was disease and denial.

This affected every aspect of my executive career. To reassure myself of my own self-worth, I'd started grinding those around me down in order to raise myself up.

I'll admit that I did enjoy routinely intimidating my two superiors and other executives I felt were weak in the company in the other divisions. Beginning with highlighting examples of underperformance in their division at my initial senior level meeting, I graduated to other ways and means of distributing my anger and anxiety around. Not returning their urgent phone calls was a big favorite. Refusing to work with many of the weaker executives in a teamwork approach to a problem was at the top of the list, especially when I could do it in front of others in a particularly hurtful way. While just another expression of my anger at my sickness, it's another point of my professional life I'm not very proud of. It only worsened the relationships. I helped nothing in doing that, especially the staff members.

I knew I was smarter than many of them were, and I let them know it daily.

I was also the same bully I denied believing I had become in grade school. I had learned nothing in more than twenty years. The only saving grace was I never transferred my abuse to any subordinate level staff, only to those at the executive level. At least from a professional point of view, they had some of it coming.

The highlight of the whole last two years with the company, in complete honesty, was the trip to Paris I earned for Abby and me to take in November 1985. France has become a very special place for us since then, and we vowed, like young couples will crazily do, to eventually get a home there.

We would do just that—twenty years later. Wasn't so "crazy" after all I guess.

But that would be another world away as I look back on it.

But by now, Joe, the old president of the original company I

worked for in very late 1979 (remember him?), now worked for
me six years and about three months later.

From the warehouse to the penthouse in six years.

I had been made the company marketing manager and
would run all company marketing as well as maintain my central division management duties. But I was already setting up
for what I thought was the future of my financial fortune.

Software. I formed my own company, Lone Star Software,
after we returned from France in December 1985. I was sure that
would lead to more money.

Wouldn't more money help end the anxiety? That had to be
a solution, I thought.

                             ●   ●

1986 mrked the lowest point of my professional career
when I had to visit a psychiatrist for the first time. For
anxiety and depression, I thought. Obviously, it wasn't.

We had begun to lay off employees for the first time in
company history. Not in my division, the central, but in both
the Houston-based southern and Dallas-based northern divisions. I was asked to take on both central and southern sales
management, where I would be made an executive and move to
Houston.

I told the president yes, but I really meant no. I never moved
or planned to move one bit. Run it from Austin or I'll be gone
was eventually the ultimatum.

The second part of the ultimatum was an eighty-seven page
business plan for our diversification of the distribution business
by building routine light-gauge, sheet-metal work ourselves
with a minimum investment of money both we and the holding
firm had. This alone would improve profitability of our number

one accessory more than 35 percent, as well as provide jobs for many of the workers we were laying off.

Being forced to needlessly lay off workers had brought me to the point where the stress level and depression were so high on my undiagnosed thyroid disease that I had now developed anxiety and depression so severe that I thought psychiatric care was needed.

Psychiatric care wasn't the solution the doctor told me after just two visits. A different job with different leadership probably was. And cut the caffeine way down.

The doctor was right.

But I still felt I *had* to find a solution for this and had spent almost eighteen hours a day on this business plan for a full month to get it prepared for the company board meeting. For some reason, I was taking this company-wide failure in sales as personal.

This was a huge mistake. I had lost my ability, once a very strong one, to separate my business life from who I was personally. I would learn to overcome that phobia before I was ultimately diagnosed. The financial markets will teach you that or break you first.

But for now, I had two ultimatums on the table for the company board meeting. Both issues were tabled for the immediate future by the president while cutbacks were discussed then subsequently ordered for me to execute.

I knew how my two supervisors would act. No way would they let me start my own division out of their control.

I resigned the next day but agreed to stay until year end: December 31, 1986.

Or until I finished the dirty work of laying off another dozen people for them.

Lone Star Software was ready to go as a business on its own by this time. A basic product had been developed to price commodity options, and Abby and I had begun to look for partner programmers to develop this product further, as well as additional products for the stock and futures markets we could add to the company's offering. From this, we hoped to father a trading and brokerage firm down the line.

I was more than glad to go; I was sure once again that it was the job that was making me sick. For certain, the leadership was.

The company I left in December 1986 went into bankruptcy about eight months into 1987, after I left. Both the president and my senior executive were terminated at that time.

# Am I Happy Yet?

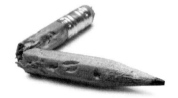

I t was a happy spring and summer after my leaving the company. Abby and I had decided that the new computer programs would have to be developed at a very slow pace to begin with. There were plenty of other issues to deal with when starting a new business. We reasoned I should take some time off for myself, just to play golf at the club and relax. Despite the stress most feel when starting a new business, it was far better on me than working at my previous job. So it's no surprise that during this time, many of my symptoms began to relax as well.

We took some small vacation trips, and I got my golf handicap down to five. That was as low as it's ever been and was good enough for a first flight club championship win at our club that summer.

We only took three more vacations in the next ten years.

My trading had gone well. The market had been rising the whole spring and summer of 1987, but I thought there was a problem with the technical reading of the market. So I began the first of my "market letters" to close friends and accounts of mine, as well as Abby's coworkers. The suggestion was to sell the stock from our investment and retirement accounts and move into the short-term cash fund. I felt a correction had to be coming soon in August 1987. The correction didn't come until October though.

I still write those letters to this day—a surprising number to the same people now as back then—but I did not get short the market at that time or recommend it. In retrospect, it was a big mistake, and one I've repeated since. But in 1987, you could not get short in almost any kind of retirement, IRA, or 401k program. We still had enjoyed a quite profitable run and, most importantly, had cashed it out.

The computer programming had also gone exceptionally well during this relaxed time. It always seemed when anxiety and related symptoms were low, productivity went up in inverse proportion. A simple version of *Option Master,* a software program I had written for the analysis of any future or commodity option that was publicly traded, was donated into what was then commonly known as the public domain, or basically a free program to anyone who cared to download or copy it. I later licensed it to a major futures exchange to be given away as an instructional and educational tool for the public. A modified Windows version of it was still being given away last year.

More and more I had gravitated away from the stock market to the commodities and futures markets because I felt the growth of foreign exchange was not only imminent but would be dramatic. It had to be. I had built the Russian oil rigs myself. This was the way of the future, I was sure. Besides, currency trading was always very exciting.

And it went on, almost twenty-four hours a day. That made it perfect for me; a new nighttime mistress was found.

The much more advanced version of *Option Master* I had written for personal use had begun to work pretty well and was highly effective in hedging situations. A *hedge* in trading terms is using the options on the actual foreign currency futures contracts to "hedge" or protect you against a sharp move against your position in the underlying contracts already held, either long or short. The pricing of currency futures options would get away from their fair value a lot during the volatile trading period from 1987 to 1990. It was my job to take advantage of that every time I could, for both myself as well as my accounts.

Quite by lucky accident, I renewed an acquaintance made during our first trip to Paris in 1985 and began to license the advanced version of the program in France to a major bank. They used it to help hedge their exchanges between French francs and Japanese yen futures—commonly called a *cross* or a *foreign cross* when it did not involve a "US dollar" side to a US futures position.

It was natural to begin licensing the program to US banks and trading departments, as well as our French, and now Mexican bank customers. However, in order to do so, the Commodity Futures Trading Commission and the National Futures Association, the regulatory agencies of the US commodity business, required you to hold at least a Series 3 license. These licenses were obtained by first being sponsored by a brokerage operation and their clearing firm, and then taking and passing a one hundred-question test, mostly on ethics and regulations, held at testing centers around the states.

I was sponsored quickly in August 1987 and then studied and passed the exam on October 4, 1987, just a few weeks before the stock market crash.

During this training period I found myself stuck at the graphics phase on the development of a new module for the option-trading program. As a result of that, I met and contracted out with two geniuses from the University of Texas named Marc and John.

They would become my partners for the next year and a half.

They had been working on a chart analysis program of their own while in college called *Trade Sight* that would perform chart-based technical analysis for any stock, bond, commodity, future, or mutual fund. They also had a version that they were developing that would work in real-time, or actually perform the analysis while the markets were trading live as each trade occurred. A fairly new idea at the time, this is now the standard in market analysis software. But more than twenty years ago, there was virtually no competition.

They quickly helped me through my simple problem, and we agreed to partner on *Trade Sight*. I would write the code for the different technical indicators, as well as write the instruction manual on how to use the software. They would focus on the graphics portion of the software—a most advanced and sophisticated one, as well as the continued development of the real-time version. We would all do marketing, but I would take the marketing show on the road with me as I began to speak at trading conferences around the US for the next two years, regarding trading foreign currency futures options and their analysis and fair value pricing, using, of course, the *Option Master* and *Trade Sight* programs.

What they commonly call now the "rubber chicken" circuit of sales and marketing.

Soon, the sixteen- to eighteen-hour days became some days without sleeping.

I felt that was just fine, normal in fact. You're supposed to be overly busy when you start your own business! Especially the first one.

And sooner or later, you enter that point where not sleeping becomes "normal" for you. Whether it's anxiety-based, health-based, workload required, or driven for success—whatever. You are not only very, very sick, if you do not get yourself under clinical care immediately, you are in *denial*.

And that usually only leads you to one location when you're sick: the cemetery plot.

It was so easy to justify then, and Abby was a good sleeper too. I could slip out of bed every night—if I even came to bed before she went to sleep—and get on the phones to see how the yen was trading in Tokyo, how interest rates were shaping up in Europe before our markets opened, or a myriad of other trading or programming details always to be done. Only to hop back to the bedroom as the alarm went off like I had just gotten up.

That's why I've always had a full-blown trading office in my home, regardless of how many offices I would have available, rented or owned. I still do.

I was an impossible liar by late year 1987, hiding my drive for success in the markets just like I would hide an affair with a mistress. But it was really the same mistress as the ones before: *money*. Only much more dangerous conduct now than ever to obtain it.

I was also entering what can become the final and fatal phase of incurable lifetime disease, complete *denial*, at that same time.

I know this as fact. After twenty-one years of denial behavior, I nearly died myself.

W hen you traded futures or commodities, up until just a few years ago, they were only traded in a "live pit," in what is commonly known as the "open auction" process. Pit traders and those upstairs in the exchange offices, as well as customers around the world, traded during consistent, regular hours the "pits" were open. Things in 1987 were much different without the Internet and the virtually twenty-four-hour trading that goes on now.

Orders had to be placed and prices returned on those same orders by phone. This is where I met one of the greatest friends of my life to this day: Tommy.

Tommy has the perfect financial business personality. He is totally understated about everything in trading. It is the only way to last over twenty years in the business.

We became the greatest of friends over the phone, sometimes five to six hours a day—almost nonstop when trading was heavy. It was almost four years later before we met in person. But how we met didn't matter to us; we were soul-mate buddies from day one. People thought it unusual to have made such a friend over the telephone alone first, but we didn't and never have.

We both began our careers in the financial business the same month—October 1987. It was a time of one of the greatest one-day crashes in the history of the stock market, and those who survived in the financial industry through that period did so by becoming a closer knit community for many years to come. We both loved the excitement involved in currency trading developing at that time. Tommy had a strong interest in the software development side of the business I was working hardest at. I had an obsession to learn a great deal more about floor operations and floor trading he conducted daily. It was a natural friendship, benefiting both from day one, that has grown to this day.

There's an old saying you've probably heard about the financial markets: "If you want a friend, get a dog." But that's not the way it really is in our business among ourselves—I bet much like it isn't in the NFL or on the PGA tour too. The financial world is just like those franchises in one sense; if you've made it to the professional level, the least you deserve from your associates and compatriots is respect. One thing that every professional who's dealt with Tommy has for him is respect.

It's been the same respectful and very helpful attitude when I've trained or been trained by other professionals. I still train with professional traders to this day to learn new and/or different trading techniques. The markets change all the time. You can never learn too much about them from those who really will teach some of what they know will work in some market situations. Thirty or more years of experience is totally worthless if you won't adapt to what's happening today. The market doesn't have a memory.

Tommy knew how to handle "hot" people, or the highly driven, type-A (diseased though I was) personalities because he handled them every day just like you or I pet and rub the family dog. The anxiety level in the commodities and futures markets is almost always way over the top. Few last more than a year or two as "locals" (people who lease a seat on the exchange in order to trade in the pits) or professional "screen" traders, who trade using analysis software on their computers in an office with live data.

Tommy lived with me for hours at a time in hope and love as I grew my business—first from the software side to the brokerage side, all the way up to the advisor stage for many years. I lived and loved with him as his mom fought her losing battle with cancer and the pain that surrounded him every day until the ultimate victory of his wedding to an unbelievable lady and the birth of an incredible daughter.

Without Tommy, I would not have survived as a professional in the financial markets. I just simply wouldn't have made it. I also wouldn't be anything near the man I am today. His innate ability to deal with highly stressed and anxious people on the floor of the various commodity exchanges every day for hours at a time was invaluable help. Working in one of the most stressful of professions around, he lifted me up by taking the edge off losing trades, low days, and routine business anxiety with a joke or example that told me he cared about what I cared about most, whatever happened.

Both my French and Mexican bank customers had begun to refer brokerage my way, so it was only natural I open my own office. In February 1988, I did just that after the usual regulatory and licensing requirements had been completed.

I now had my own software company, a partnered software company, and a privately held brokerage operation within a year and a half of starting my own business.

Only one thing was left: to become the equivalent of a mutual fund manager in the commodities business, or what is known as a CTA or Commodity Trading Advisor, generally considered the elite of the elite in the world of commodity futures trading.

I would complete that process, including the production of my actual track record of trading and hedging, to be legally recognized by the necessary regulatory agencies on August 11, 1988.

That year I was listed in "Who's Who" in *Futures Magazine,* an honor I would enjoy for every year until I sold the business.

We had a terrific party after the article came out, and my partner Marc, while enjoying a glass of champagne, remarked, "Wow, man, you've got to be happy about things now!"

I naturally laughed aloud. "Yeah, baby." But that wasn't the truth at all.

I wasn't happy. Not at all. And it felt like something was gaining on me.

I was going to have to work harder.

* *

I had worked hard and had made some money, but you would have had to be blind to not see the Windows platform coming as the dominant software issue in America in early 1990. I thought so, and I thought our run in both software and trading was nearing an end. We had had a great run and had made some good calls on market direction and some better hedges.

Like any other trader, I had made some stinking bad trades too—plenty of them. That's just the way it goes in this business. I have managed to never carry what professionals call "baggage" around with them in the form of remembering bad trades or big losers.

Not only did I know it was wrong to do this, but my ego by then was bigger than Canada, probably approaching the size of the Pacific Ocean.

I had read that Coach Vince Lombardi always said his Packers never "lost" a game; the clock just ran out on them. I had always felt the same about my trading, hedging, and advising; I was never wrong, just early.

There was another reason I knew that selling out was right around the corner for the business I had built up. Abby had caught me lying about my sleep and workload. You can't lie forever to someone you live with. It's stupid and impossible.

And she had given me the closest thing to an ultimatum she has ever done before or since. "Stop the trading business and slow down, or I'll be forced to leave your side. I won't watch you kill yourself while you refuse to listen to reason," she told me. So it was time for a change, and maybe a good rest too. Abby was more important than anything, including money.

We were lucky to find willing buyers for all businesses before the mini-recession of 1991 to 1993. We got top dollar for the brokerage, software, and management businesses from three different corporate buyers.

The symptoms list had gone ballistic now. Inability to sleep more than a few hours at a time, if ever. Skin breakdowns again, this time all the way up to the face and chest, which had required my wife, who had joined a medical manufacturer in 1985, to get the hydrocortisone cream *by the case* from medical distributors so I could hide the problem. The lack of my ability to control my body temperature was hitting a new low, and I had lost forty pounds. I explained the weight loss away to all by attributing it to an extreme exercise program I was on.

I was rail thin and looked sick. Probably because I was.

But I could smell another opportunity coming: the RTC, or the Resolution Trust Corporation.

And we had a little cash money on hand. How convenient!

•  •

I began by buying small parcels of residential land from the Resolution Trust Corp., holding them for a while as the area stabilized or most of the previously available lots were bought out. During that time, Abby and I would clean them up and trim trees and shrubs so they would show as a property much better. I only bought the cheapest lots in the most expensive areas of town.

I had battles with large builder groups on virtually every deal I made. I was always "cherry picking" the best value lots when their brokers had made deals for large or entire groups of lots in a good subdivision, inevitably including the one I wanted to buy. But Abby and I were cash buyers, and to the RTC that came first. A hard cash, no financing offer with a thirty-day closing date could beat out almost every large builder group we competed with. RTC wanted to show action on properties rather than potential deals.

I started buying inexpensive and proven previously built house plans from home plan magazines that would fit on small and non-traditional-sized lots. I would then package these with the lot as a turnkey package, where the buyer could get not only a single family home lot but a building plan that would fit within the confines of the local permit process and, of course, the lot itself.

It went very well.

After less than six months on any property, I had returns of between 25 to 40 percent on relatively small investments diversified out around the best subdivisions of Austin. It was a great business. The only problem was that the inventory was drying up. RTC would wind up being out of residential properties of any value by early 1992.

We talked it over night after night and figured the only thing left was to switch to commercial. There was still plenty of commercial inventory left, and what had not sold already was or was about to be reduced again. And this time we decided we would develop it ourselves. No flipping. Another real company. And one that would have a philanthropic goal portion to it now as well.

Several years before, when I had begun the financial software business, I had begun to do radio for the blind through the Texas School for the Blind. I did this, off and on, for more than fifteen years with a program called "Dollars and Sense." The show had grown in scope quite a bit over that time, and Abby joined me in the program after about ten years to occasionally interject the point of view of nonprofessional investment questions and comments. We also began to interview prominent blind people in the central Texas area about their success and how they overcame their challenges. We met and worked with some wonderful people who had overcome a great deal in their lives to become successful.

We would make a financial goal component of the new business to help the blind, as well as the Presbyterian Church with a portion of profits. However long it took. This was important to us because we wanted to give back to the community we lived in, not just take from it. If we could put something into the community from our profits, we were sure it would benefit all. I secretly hoped it would help me feel better too.

The only promise: I wouldn't work like I had before. I swore that repeatedly.

Then I broke that promise for fifteen more years. Lying *all* the time to every friend and most important person in my life almost every day. No different than before. Worse.

The same old liar, just more cagey and more aware than ever now of the mistakes you make while in hiding.

I was sure I could handle it. I had actually begun getting better again by now. Real estate development was a breeze compared to foreign currency futures trading and hedging.

And besides, wasn't this really for charity too?

I was beyond disease, self-abuse, and denial by this time. I was now lying to myself.

•  •

The residential land deals had been a healing time of low stress and relatively little anxiety for me. We never had to go all in or take large risks on anything to do these little deals.

That would change. It has to if you're going to really financially grow as a small business.

We hadn't been able to find a decent self-storage facility for the new boat we had purchased to try to help put some fun back in our life a little more than a year earlier. We had both come to love boating, water skiing, and just relaxing off the back of the boat. And in contrast to my other interests, like golf and investing, we could do it together. But the facilities available to us to store our boat didn't seem managed well, and we laughed because we might have an opportunity. Then true to Abby's pragmatic style, she said, "Joke's over; why keep looking? Let's build our own. We know what we want is what everybody else wants." I had to admit I felt she was right.

I had been investing in self-storage limited partnerships for several years but had never operated, much less owned, a storage facility. But neither of us ever thought that would be a problem. We would just run the business the way we wanted a boat and self-storage place to be run if we were the customers.

In all honesty, as simple as it sounds, it has been a very good business philosophy for almost fourteen years. One we still maintain today.

But just building your own storage facility always seems so easy. I can't tell you how many times I have had people tell me they were going to do it. But it's not easy to get a business built from the ground up, especially if you have to personally borrow and act as general contractor yourself.

But Abby and I agreed this was the time in our lives to try it, if ever. The fantastic commercial parcel we had located we could buy for cash and install the utilities to. But we would have to go all-in again with all the cash we had for the second time in our lives.

I didn't have a doubt, but I knew the symptoms would be back like an obnoxious relative, probably worse than ever.

I justified that was just the price that would have to be paid for something as important as this project was. There was always an anxiety price I had to pay for anything that wasn't routine or a new challenge. I simply didn't know that both the noticeable and invisible health issues consistently reemerging during stressful times were the exact symptoms that thyroid, metabolic, and anxiety-based diseases mimic: allergies, arthritis, anger, anxiety, skin problems, moodiness, temperature-control issues, excess sweating, irritable bowels, worsening vision, weight gain and loss, fatigue, depression, and inability to concentrate or focus, among so many others many of us suffer.

Each symptom can be attributed to something other than a serious thyroid, metabolic, or clinical anxiety disease. That's the ultimate paradox in getting the proper diagnosis. I lump these diseases together many times in this book because I've learned that many of the treatments are as similar as the symptoms are. It sure makes it easy not only to misdiagnose but to deny as well.

In any case, all three are medical problems, not the mental problems I had feared so long. Thyroid, metabolic, and clinical anxiety sufferers need a medical doctor. We must start there if we want our health to improve.

I just wasn't going to accept the fact that I needed to get started with a doctor. I had been lying to everybody I knew, as well as myself, for so long that my problems had started to seem natural, even routine. And I had become exceptionally adept at fooling my wife and close friends into believing the same thing.

It was really dumb luck my denial and justification hadn't cost me my life or my marriage by this time.

•  •

I had produced a business plan for a limited partnership to build out around one-third of the first commercial property we owned in three distinct phases. After holding meetings with potential local limited partners, I decided to try to borrow the money ourselves, even if Abby and I would have to personally guarantee the loan, which we ultimately had to do. You almost always have to with your first big commercial deal.

It was much better than dealing with a large group of amateur partners. And ultimately, far, far more profitable.

The partnership document was very useful in the loan process, and I met another life-changing friend, Dan, in the late spring of 1994. Dan was a bank officer and commercial lender at a very aggressive and entrepreneurial local branch of a bank that actually had its headquarters located in west Texas. He had had a great wealth of experience in the banking business. He'd held every post from examiner to bank officer. Dan is the ultimate in the old school of "deal judges" that bankers really used to be. This was especially important in the smaller community-type banks, and even more so when their branches were hundreds of miles from their executive offices. The executives *really* relied on the opinions of the local officers.

He wasn't the first banker I approached, but he was the best banker I had met. I knew this immediately when I met him. Quiet confidence is a great asset, one which Dan enjoys a great deal of. I call him the gentle giant. He's about six feet five inches tall and played quarterback and fullback on scholarship for the University of Texas Longhorns. I can tell you with confidence he's one tough guy. But you wouldn't know it from the way his wife and daughter wrap him around their fingers.

He took a personal interest in the project from day one, I think partially because we were immediately beset by the worst luck you could have in the development business.

The bad luck began by running into a local building inspector, who was involved in the permit process at length, who told me in great detail that he routinely "worked for everybody who builds around here," meaning the small but growing suburb of Austin we were located in.

I had grown up building and rebuilding more than self-storage facilities, and I informed the inspector I would take care of my own subcontractors and we would never waste his time by calling for an inspection that I personally had not gone over the work completed. If errors were made in the construction so serious as to fail a legitimate code issue, we would take care of the routine reinspection fees that are paid to a municipality to cover anytime a mistake is made, usually a miscommunication of what is local code.

But I didn't get his message. I was too naïve. He wanted on the payroll. *My payroll.*

Otherwise, my building plans awaiting preliminary approval and processing to the next step, the civil engineer the municipality used to approve the drainage and water control issues, could be delayed. And at this time, unfortunately, my plans were delayed. They would be delayed until he was paid off, either as an inspector or just under the table; either way, the plans weren't going past his hands until he got cash.

I immediately called Dan for a meeting. We met the next day in his office. I told him flat-out what I was up against. He and I agreed expressly, without hesitation, *we wouldn't pay.* I guess we really became much better friends right then, as well as business associates.

I also learned the value of total honesty in a tough situation. It was too bad I couldn't apply those same principles in the rest of my life.

Anger had come back again, the kind that would last a while. I wouldn't be shaken down. That inspector would have to be exposed and then broken.

But in retrospect, it would have been faster, and cheaper, to just pay him off. I hate to admit it to you, but that's the way it often is. It's an important lesson I've been forced to learn. As it was, we hired the biggest and nastiest lawyers in Austin. It took five months additional delay, and several thousand dollars, but that inspector was gone. Our permits had moved quickly to the safety department. The civil engineering was perfect.

Only to find problem two. The fire department only had one-hundred-foot fire hoses!

Our building site was four hundred feet deep by more than three hundred and fifty feet wide. That meant thirty thousand extra dollars over budget just for fire hydrants that, to this day—fourteen years later—thank goodness have never been used.

Now I had to go back to Dan again because that was out of our budget. He understood. You have to understand when you're a decision-making professional in his position I guess. Dan had more development experience than I did in reality. He knew what could happen—anything. Nobody else could build the size we were building without the unknown fire safety issue covered anyway. The municipalities in and around Austin were as tough to build in then as they are today, which is to say, they are some of the toughest development regulations of any community in the country. There was simply no way around this unknown, but unlucky, problem.

But one hundred feet of hose per fire truck! You have got to be kidding me. Who could have imagined a thirty thousand dollars extra expense for that? I never did.

It hurt financially, and obviously, I've never forgotten it either. But over time you learn to just accept that those things happen in commercial development and get with the construction. That's what really matters. You can't earn any income until the project is open.

With that blind side covered, I was sure we had it made and were on track now. All that was left was final approval from the city council. The final piece of bad luck was they decided they didn't want a phase project on what was already becoming the city's main thoroughfare. They wanted a much larger commitment up front. More than 65 percent of the project had to be built to begin with. That was double our 33 percent. It would make us almost double the construction loan as well. Their decision was final. And a legal challenge would have cost tens of thousands, even fifteen years ago.

Back once more to Dan again. The new problem was that

we were going to be forced to both build and, of course, borrow more than ever planned. Period.

He never blinked. It was the truth, and he knew it, and we had been through too much by then to even consider quitting on this deal. Something this hard just had to be worth it.

"Okay, we'll get it done," was all he said.

And we did, finally closing a loan eleven months after the original, smaller loan was approved. We closed for almost double the original loan amount and more than double the original size of development, with a bonanza of fire hydrants to go along.

For what it's worth, in my opinion, to have any chance at success in your first commercial development, you *must* have a banker that's more than just experienced, or you may have no chance at all to make it. The failure probably won't be due to anything you've done or not done or could predict. It's not what you know that kills your deals.

The breakdowns in business occur almost always due to the unknown and impossibly unexpected. It's the same trying to live as normal, in denial, with any unknown or undiagnosed lifelong incurable disease. It will always cause an unexpected breakdown the same way. The big difference is it doesn't just kill a business deal, it can kill the sufferer.

I had done my lender homework and worked hard, but I knew I had gotten lucky, really lucky, in meeting Dan. I shudder to think where I'd be without him now.

I had always run my business life very squarely, near perfection, and have faced down two IRS audits where I actually received very small refunds after a total business review. It was too bad I couldn't perform nearly as well on a personal basis.

But you can't when you're always lying or covering up something, whether it's sickness or anxiety. It doesn't matter.

And the symptoms began to reappear with ferocity in our groundbreaking month of July 1995. The anxiety caused by borrowing more money than anybody I knew had borrowed to build the business caused me to drop to my lowest adult weight during the construction period. Unable to sleep for days, I was constantly in anger and anxiety as the interest rate clock ticked on.

I'd now passed the lying to myself phase and completed passage into the justification portion of my denial. Beginning with thinking that I'm just able to work harder than others will only last so long. It's easy to accept that philosophy at first, but soon you realize after a few years of experience it's much more difficult to achieve. There are a whole lot of hard workers out there, and they aren't sick, just motivated.

I was more than motivated; I was starting to know inside I must be sick. I knew I needed to get to a doctor and find out what was wrong. This anger, anxiety, and myriad of other symptoms couldn't keep going on forever unless something was really wrong.

But my ego held me back. I mean, could I still be known as Superman if I had a bunch of health problems?

●  ●

Actually, the delays in not opening in 1994 had not hurt as much as we thought possible; plus, the economy was just turning up strongly in 1995, our opening year. For sure, many had worked hard to get the project up and running, but it's also very helpful to have good timing. Our timing had been very good and, as with such things, a bit lucky too.

We started renting units from day one and showed straight up growth for seven consecutive years.

During this period of solid business growth, in 1997 we built a beautiful two-story custom home. I had purchased the basic design prints back during our RTC days in 1991. It was in one of the most desirable parts of town known as Westlake Hills. It was a tough lot but almost one-half acre, and I knew I could make it work. We finally struck a cash deal for the land and began right away. No crooked inspector this time. It was county authorities, so I hired a bureaucratic specialist to help, and permits went fast.

We worked hand in hand with the carpenter to modify the house exactly the way we wanted it, inside and out. Cherry hardwood floors, hand-built double staircase with chandeliers at the critical points. It was a beautiful home I had built in large measure myself, including designing and building the fifteen-hundred-square-foot outdoor deck.

I'll never forget the day Dan and his family came to visit the home at a small party. He told me, "When I build a home, you're going to build it for me!" It was a great compliment from a man from whom a compliment like that meant an awful lot. But like so many of us with problems, all I could see were the imperfections in the home I'd built, a mirror image of the imperfections I felt about my own life. In such a mind-set, it's almost impossible to grasp the positive about anything achieved or accomplished.

Was I happy yet? *No.* There's more than ever to do now with another mortgage.

*I have to work harder,* I thought. Another cycle of anxiety and symptoms would start again with the addition of a new financial responsibility. I knew they'd come before they began, but I was sure I could keep hiding them.

● ●

In late 2001 when the highway was improved in front of our business, our entrance was blocked for fourteen months. We hadn't suffered that much from the stock market decline and minor recession of 2001 and 2002. People are always moving during such times. But the highway blockage hurt our business more than any competition could, so we reinvested in additional RV storage land and improved our street appeal with a totally remodeled business office. Within a few months, after the highway was finished, we were near 100-percent occupancy again. And profits were higher than ever.

Things had gone pretty well for several years in a health sense too. My symptoms were recurring, but not as badly as during the stress of trading. By now I could definitely tell some symptoms were triggered by stress-type events, and some were not.

I was more confused about myself than ever, but I would be damned if I'd show it, much less go see a doctor, even if one had become my friend like Doc Mike had.

I had begun trading again, but very quietly, and no night-time or currency markets. No hiding it from Abby either. I had her approval and just kept it in perspective. Stocks and some options. A few bonds too. Not much for somebody like me, and that's at least one promise I've kept since I made it. No over-work trading. I swore it to her, and I've kept true to it.

One redeeming promise kept at least. But it was and is something to build on.

2003 was a good rebound year, for both the markets and our business, which had seen further expansion again. Abby and I began to want a different place for our final "tree house" home. By now, we had both realized that building in what we had once thought of as the best part of town had now seemed to become the most snobbish part of town, and we had made a bit of a mistake. No matter how beautiful and impressive the home was, neither of us was ever happy in that area of Austin. We didn't fit in. Or maybe, it was more like I didn't fit in. The truth is that Abby can fit in anywhere.

So with the stock market and occupancy profits having gone to record levels, we noted real estate, especially acreage properties, were very still very soft in price. We looked at a lot of good potential properties, and even more stinkers, for months before we found forty unspoiled tree-covered acres of pine and oak twenty-five minutes from the airport. A cash deal cut the price a further 20 percent, and we owned it less than sixty days after seeing it.

We would start the guesthouse of our future estate right away.

Abby was ecstatic. That kind of accomplishment should make anyone happy. Except, of course, someone who was pretty sick like I was.

It shocked me some at the new feelings after the purchase. I had never had second thoughts about taking on any project, large or small, but I was suddenly feeling a new anxiety, one that made me suspect that I might have bitten off more than I could chew. That was a new sensation for me, and I guess I realize now that a sudden lack of confidence exhibited as depression and irritability was settling in at a very extreme level. Another new feeling that was both bothersome and unexpected was that I was starting to feel tired—a brand new symptom. But one that almost every single thyroid disease sufferer will eventually face, regardless of the exact nature of their disease.

But that was impossible, I told myself. I never got tired; in my whole life I had never gotten tired.

*I'm just getting old!* I laughed to myself.

But I told everybody else, including Doc Mike, nothing like the truth at all.

Are you kidding?

      •    •

The stock market had been moving at a terrific pace for years now, both up and down. Traders like I am don't care if the market goes up or down, just that it goes. I just need movement to make money. And I had begun to donate some portion of the profits to the church for several years. I usually took them a check right before Christmas in person.

The Christmas of 2004 was a good check, like the year had been. This wasn't our annual stewardship pledge; this was a yearly gift of devotion from what I'd been able to earn, if any, out of the markets. To show you the great love Jim, who was senior pastor at that time at our church in Austin, had for me, when I brought the annual check to the church in hand as usual, I ran into Jim on the stairs up to the business offices. I winked and told him with some measure of gleeful pride that I had brought a "good one" this year, but he honestly could have cared less how much money I gave and never even opened the envelope I had busted my butt all year trading to bring.

He only wanted to know and cared about how *I* was doing then.

Forget it if you think you're fooling your pastor—if you have one—and you're sick. Especially if they've gotten to know you at all. Few are that good at lying. I obviously hadn't been, and believe me, I had become a *good* liar.

Jim's probing questions had bothered me. He was more than a biblical scholar; he was an expert at reading people, and he probed me for several minutes in couched manner about depression, anxiety, and my understanding that his love and care for me was not based on how I gave but on who I was. I had to get to see Doc Mike pretty soon. There were just too many things wrong for too long now. And if Jim suspected, others might as well. For those of us in hiding, denial, or justification, that's tantamount to disaster.

Abby and I had also started talking seriously about *our* health for some months too. I wasn't fooling her anymore either. She knew some things were wrong, but at least she held back from calling me the outright liar I was. She also couched it in terms of "our" health to keep my enormous ego at bay. Abby had always been more than just beautiful.

So right before I gave Jim that Christmas check, I wired funds from the stock account to the French *notaire* (title agent) to purchase a town home in the tiny village of Ecueille' we had just visited during our twenty-first anniversary trip that previous November 2004, our Christmas present for each other that year.

Nineteen years to the month after we dreamed together of doing this on our first visit to France in November 1985, we signed a deal to close on a hundred-year-old home near the very center of France in November 2004. In fact, the region is known as *Centre*. It's about two hours south of Paris by train, a little more by car.

This *had* to make me happy now! I was absolutely sure of it.

We knew the little house needed a good deal of work and to have the third floor finished, but we also had decided neither of us was going to live forever. Better to enjoy some things now than always saving for the next deal or retirement, we had both agreed.

I had honestly been feeling better lately too. Things had been going super right up until January 27, 2005.

That was the day of the wreck.

And I still wasn't really happy all the way I should have been and wasn't going to be either after this coming experience for a very long time—in fact, until I was positively diagnosed almost exactly four years later.

⬤　⬤

That Thursday of January 27, 2005, was a rainy day but only moderately cold. Usually in Austin, January is kind of the rainy season, and we don't get that many days at or below freezing. It had been much colder the day before, and the rain had made the roads slicker than usual. I decided to get out of the office a little sooner than my habit. I could finish my trading at my home office, and our office manager had things under control.

The lady in the SUV passed me just as I left my office then took a street which can cut off waiting at a long light just a few hundred feet from the intersection. The street has since been closed due to the many accidents from people trying to cut around traffic. I noted she had her daughter with her in the front seat, and she seemed to be driving way too fast for the conditions.

The 2004 E-class Mercedes I drove was bought not only to satisfy my always growing ego, but Abby and I had checked it out as a very safe car.

Good thing. It didn't break up after a double t-bone collision. I think most cars would.

I saw the lady's face and her daughter's face right before they hit me after running the stop sign that was used to block people from cutting off the heavy traffic corner. That impact would have never hurt me because all the airbags went off.

She fled the scene immediately and was arrested trying to get her car fixed by a body shop about a hundred miles away a couple of months later. She was driving on a suspended license without insurance.

The real problem was that her large vehicle at high speed easily knocked me through the grass median, which was slick as ice by the rain all day, and right into the opposite lane of traffic. The road has a sixty-five-mile-per-hour speed limit.

The heavy truck that hit me next hit me with all my airbags going down and no protection at all. And he was going the speed limit: sixty-five.

I don't remember the second impact, probably because when it happened, the laptop I had always carried for trading purposes was just lying on the passenger front seat. It hit my head so hard the rebound took it up and broke through the *closed* sunroof. They found it about sixty feet away. It's not a good idea to leave a laptop computer loose in your passenger front seat.

That was how I got the skull fracture. I was out for about fifteen to eighteen minutes according to the paramedics, maybe more. But that wasn't the worst part in my opinion, even though it would bring on vertigo for some months and give me a pretty hard time.

The worst part for me was the three broken ribs and collapsed right lung. Not just the pain of the ribs, but the hiccups you constantly get as your lung tries to reinflate. I can honestly tell you, I have never known pain like having hiccups with three broken ribs.

I can share with you how to get rid of hiccups quickly if you don't already know. Take a full glass of water, and tilt your head back as far as you can, hold your nose, and drink without stopping. Even if a hiccup makes you stop a second, drink constantly. You can then belch the hiccups away very quickly. If I hadn't learned that trick, I probably would have started considering suicide.

There were plenty of other injuries as well: to my back, obviously, torn ligaments in the right knee, and the worst bruises of my life on my torso and at the hip from the strain of the double collisions against the seatbelt restraints. I guess it was better to have had those than to have been thrown out of the car like the laptop was.

I came to while they were treating me through the broken window as the firemen had begun using the jaws of life to pry the door open. They told me they had my wife on the phone of the paramedic. They had already told her they believed I would live, despite the severity, but they were either calling the Starflight emergency helicopter or taking me to the closest hospital, which was less than two miles away. Which did we prefer?

I told them, "Damn sure no Starflight. That costs about ten thousand! Just take me home."

Leave it to Clay to worry about the money while the paramedics are putting the EKG sensors on him to make sure he doesn't die on them at the scene. But I'm no idiot, and I could see the concern on his face and his actions. I said, "Take me to Doc Mike."

Severe head and multiple internal injuries. Forget taking me home, and it was too far to Doc Mike's offices in their opinion, so it was the hospital.

And, of course, stress like that brought every symptom I had to a new level within a few weeks. My dry skin and dandruff had hit really new heights, with sores developing on my scalp from the still unknown vitamin A deficiency. The combination of pain and anger would cause me to fly into anger, many times a rage, at the slightest mistake around me by anyone. My anxiety had grown to the point of minor panic attacks, both by having trouble breathing in a routine manner and by believing I was in the beginning stages of a heart attack. It turned out that these symptoms indeed were part of the problem, but in addition, I was not oxygenating properly due to the collapsed lung.

So that was it, not anxiety. Superman doesn't have anxiety, just a collapsed lung. Not only disease in full bloom but now denial as well.

The symptoms just weren't high enough, or without rationale, for me to do anything about them yet, and besides, I had to deal with all the rehab first. I had more excuses ready if that one weakened. I always did. Many of the injuries, especially head injuries like I had, have symptoms that are similar in nature to my thyroid disease. Things like occasional disorientation and dizziness, nausea, weight changes, depression, anxiety, irritability, and fatigue are routine symptoms people experience with head and brain injuries. I had learned that years ago from my old roommate, Jeff.

I've learned they're also routine symptoms of thyroid disease sufferers.

In reality, all I could think of, and did think of, was getting back to work, or rather, getting back to making money.

Because I knew I had to do something special then. Something not for myself or my business or even for Abby. And I knew it was going to take some serious money to do it. More than we had ever given.

A new church, one we would donate in Abby's grandparents' names, near the acreage guesthouse we already had under construction. We knew we would live there eventually, and there had never been a Presbyterian church in this whole county immediately east of Austin we would surely soon be living in.

If all the success, money, and influence I'd obtained until then hadn't really made me happy, I knew this would.

I honestly believed so at the time.

My life had been spared now twice. I had to do something. Abby agreed.

A lot of the parts of this new, seemingly impossible goal were based on her ideas.

• •

Abby took me to France to close on our house in a wheelchair.

It was a humbling experience in that wheelchair almost constantly during the trip. I'll never forget it. Until you've had to do something like that, you have no idea how tough it is for the people who are permanently bound in one. I know I didn't.

I'm sure the humbling was much needed, but the trip was heavily advised against.

But I have *never* not delivered on a deal, and I wasn't going to start, especially with the French people. We would be the first and, until just lately, the only Americans in that village. I couldn't possibly have allowed a closing date to be missed because I was hurt. It was more than just ego to me. I felt we were representing America a little bit too. I know those feelings today as ultimately being the right ones, as we have done more and more business with the French over the years since.

We met another guardian angel in France, Simone. Simone has become our combination interpreter, general contractor for the home renovation, banking and insurance agent, decorator, and perhaps most of all, loving friend, one as close to us as any of our family members. One thing we learned from her and many new friends we've made in France is that the French really do highly value overcoming adversity, and our relationship with many, including our new neighbors in the village, got off to the best of starts despite the fact I couldn't even walk or remember much of the language due to my head injury.

Simone took over our home renovation and managing the artisans (French for skilled contractors) like she was born to it. The complete renovation began immediately. She eventually became known by her subcontractors as "Madame Nazi." A match truly made in heaven. She's our kind of lady for sure.

We made it back okay, but that was one tough trip. I don't know if I could do it again. But no sense whining about it. Once I've given my word to a deal, I've got to keep it. Besides, I had learned long ago nothing any good was ever easy, especially for me.

And by now, fatigue, anxiety, and pain were starting to seem normal.

Just like lying about them did.

●  ●

My recovery was slow; as so often happens, hidden problems pop up after such physical trauma like a bad car wreck. Abby had to wind up finishing the guesthouse, taking my place as the general contractor. The vertigo had me lying in bed with my eyes closed, on the phone with the contractor, usually in Spanish, and then Abby, in English, trying to get to the bottom of whatever problem existed and come up with a solution. I could not drive for months.

The thyroid disease symptoms were growing past any point they had been in my life with the combination of stress from both the new home construction as well as the stress of the pain from the wreck. Right at the same time in life as my mom had it, severe weight change visited me as well. I freaked out the same way and went into a fanatic exercise routine, even though I wasn't supposed to yet.

Of course, this made things worse—a vicious cycle, like a rat on a treadmill.

I gained eleven pounds in one week, even though I was still bed bound and only eating some soup each day. The weight roller coaster, once started in full bloom like my disease had blossomed to, would be a nightmare that would continue until my positive diagnosis and proper treatment began nearly four years later.

Joint pain had begun to be a very serious problem too. At first, I attributed this to the extra exercise I was doing and the increased weight I was carrying. But it got too severe, and I asked Doc Mike for the first of three arthritis specialist referrals. Every time the tests came back, they were negative. Every time I left a new arthritis doctor's office, all I could say to myself was "idiots!" But I didn't have arthritis. I had thyroid disease; it was just a relatively new symptom for me but common for others.

Coming out of hiding is not easy. Don't expect it to be if you have some problems.

This is one of the main reasons, in my opinion, that such a great number of people are sick but undiagnosed today. Like I've done, for all my life now, I've never given my physician the whole ugly truth, despite the fact that my doctor was now a good friend, golf buddy, and somebody whom I knew I could trust. I was still in hiding, especially from him, because he was really, really smart.

So I would go in and say, "Doc, send me to the arthritis guy. My joints are killing me."

And he would because he trusted me and was trying to help me. But I wasn't treating him fairly back in return because I never gave him *all* the symptoms at once and let him go to work on it like a case. I made the situation impossible for him.

Especially with Doc Mike, who is a brilliant doctor, somebody I knew had the type of personality to stay on something till he found it like a bulldog does. He had spent eighteen years trying to find a cure for muscular dystrophy for goodness's sake!

But twenty-five years or more of hiding, denial, and justification are tough habits to break. But I had come way past the point possible to stop myself from these habits without specific medical treatment. It was impossible to get the treatment necessary due to the lack of a correct diagnosis. The lack of a correct diagnosis was the responsibility of many, myself of course, but also several previous doctors' misdiagnoses. This untenable circle spawned an ever-widening cycle of frustration and anger that left me nowhere to go but to begin questioning my sanity again with vigor.

Nevertheless, make no mistake about it, when it came to the anxiety issue, I stayed in hiding. I also stayed anxious. I had to; I was untreated.

The symptoms leveled off in early 2006, with a thirty-eight-pound unexplained weight gain. I was working out four to five days a week for nearly an hour and a half at a time to train my legs for an upcoming golf trip to Scotland with Dan. I ate only very small meals at night. I had begun to be sick every morning again anyway. Neither my wife nor I could explain the weight, especially in light of the exercise. I was also working frantically on the acreage property, which was always very physical work. We rededicated ourselves that year to getting the land for the gift of the church.

We purchased a little over seven acres on the most major highway in the area, which is also the airport highway, directly across from a luxury resort for cash. We subdivided almost three full acres for the new church and left the rest for a conventional office warehouse development we have created a partnership for.

I had asked a close friend, and principal of his own architectural firm, Herman, to father a small foundation to make the gift with both Abby and myself in a strictly hands off position. We would not be on the board of the foundation we would fund, nor have any interest, voting or otherwise on its actions. But the foundation would have a strong stick to use with the Presbyterian church. Herman and his hand-selected board of directors would control the gift, how and when it was made, and if necessary, whom to.

It's really quite difficult to establish a charitable foundation, we all ultimately learned. We were so fortunate to have a friend like Herman, who also strongly believed in what we were doing, because so few can get through the maze of red tape and bureaucracy of the process. But Herman managed to do it. It took us more than fifteen months though.

In December 2007, just before Christmas, Herman, Abby, and I met with our regular title agent we had been using for more than twenty years and formally gave the property to the foundation. It had cost us a whole lot more than we thought—almost a quarter of a million, virtually the same amount we started the business with twelve years before. But we all still felt it was more than worth it.

We called Dan and several other friends who had supported us in so many ways to let them know it was finally done.

And for a few weeks in early 2008, I really was happy. I was sure I'd be feeling better soon.

●　●

I knew I couldn't build the church right away. We simply didn't have enough money left to give for a decent building. It didn't matter anyway.

The Presbyterian Church USA didn't want the land. They just wanted the foundation to give it to them so they could sell it for cash. They couched the phrases slightly softer, but it was the truth. I emailed Herman briefly about how we felt about that kind of attitude when he copied me on the formal response but did not offer any alternatives. We knew both Presbyterian churches we had attended in Austin had begun on land of less than one acre, and this was almost a full three, but it wasn't good enough for the church's ruling body. "Just give us the money; we know better what to do," was basically the answer.

I don't know what Herman and the foundation have done with the land, if anything, as I write this in the spring of 2009. We don't talk about it. It's a truly blind foundation. There still is nothing on the land now. I doubt there will be until the foundation builds it, maybe for another congregation.

It was heartbreaking to me at first what had happened. But I guess you can never be too surprised at what people will do, and churches are built and run by people, not God. Both Abby and I knew it wasn't *his* fault. I had had similar bad experiences with church politics while serving on the session of Presbyterian churches as a ruling elder.

I have to say I wasn't totally surprised. I don't think Abby was either. Disappointed beyond belief, yes, but she wasn't shocked or surprised any more than I was.

In any case, the final result for me was that I had to put depression back on the symptoms list again and move it straight to the head of the line.

I was also anxious and unhappy as at anytime in my life. But it would get worse, much worse, before it got better.

# The Blowout

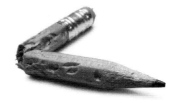

Iknew that look on Abby's face when I walked in the house, even though I'd only seen it a couple of times in more than twenty-five years. I knew it meant disaster.

We had just returned home from her special birthday celebration and our combined twenty-fifth wedding anniversary party held with our closest friends at the local Benihanna. The chef had put on a fantastic display, and the whole group was having a blast watching the onion volcano, trying to catch flying shrimp in our mouths off the knife of the chef. We had the whole works. It had been one of the best times my wife and I had had out in weeks.

Unusually, we had had to come and return home in separate cars because of work schedules, and due to an accident she just missed, I was several minutes behind.

She had only been home about ten minutes before me, but that had been enough. She had taken the call.

After so long together, Abby knew I wouldn't want her to dance around something like this with me. She told me in the strongest, straightest possible way she could, "I don't know any other way to tell you this, baby, than LeAnn's just called, and Marcia's dead."

My sister, lifetime guardian angel, and protector was dead. That news, coming on the emotional high of one of the best parties I had been to in months. A party held not only to celebrate our twenty-fifth anniversary but also mostly held for somebody I love more than anything. On the eve of a very special trip to our recently renovated home in central France that had been planned for over a year. You can imagine all the excitement that comes and builds with something like that. Then this news.

Nothing could ever hurt me like that, I thought. Nothing. But something hit me right then like nothing had ever hit me before in my entire life.

In the next few minutes I was told by the police that it was, and still is as I write today, undetermined if it was foul play or suicide, but it very much appeared to be a suicide even though my brother-in-law was a person of interest. A small caliber pistol, deep in the throat, no teeth broken, no defensive wounds, no forced entry into the home, the police were sure it was suicide. It made no sense at all to me either way. I could only think, over and over, *She is dead,* and being a pragmatist at heart, I knew without illusion this was simply the end of her tragically emotional, poor time on this earth. I had lost a most important piece of my life.

I immediately prayed, after I hung up the phone with the police, that she had finally found some desperately needed peace in the end and that heaven would be the beginning of real happiness for her.

And that was the beginning of the end and the end of the beginning of a lot of things for me too, even though I didn't know it at the time.

But outwardly, and visibly to my wife Abby, who was surely the one person in the whole world I couldn't let see me become weak, anxious, or lacking total confidence at an impossible time, I had to keep up the same old performance. I mean, after all, hadn't I been Superman for more than twenty-five years now?

I pretended to be quite calm while she cried and grieved in my arms. It was simply doing and acting like the charade artist

I had become, living and breathing as a different person for so many years now, for everybody around me, including my wife.

So as usual, I just shoved that pain right back down my throat, and I gagged on it.

I was convinced I could eat this grief too. I'd had years and years of experience at this. All that practice can make you awfully good at this sort of idiotic behavior.

But this time the pain just wasn't going to stay down.

I simply didn't know how sick I'd gotten and was still getting.

•  •

We left for our twenty-fifth anniversary trip to our home in France, literally from the funeral parlor. I had arranged a lot of special little things for Abby and me, including a stay at a five-star private hotel in the Sancerre region of France and some extra nights in Paris before we returned with a final evening dinner at our favorite restaurant in the world, *Lasserre*. All of these things had been timed out pretty exhaustively months in advance.

Except I didn't know in advance to make time for grief too.

I did my best to hide my sadness and sickness, doing a pretty good job most of the time I thought. We really did have a great anniversary trip, despite the circumstances.

Only to return to a stock market crash.

It definitely looked like one before we left, but I had been out of almost all long positions, even in our retirement accounts, since the market letter I wrote in June 2007 calling for a top very soon from a technical standpoint. I had received some rather angry responses from that letter, and I had indeed missed the top in price by about two hundred Dow Jones Index points and about two and a half months time. So few, if any, had made changes to their accounts. Now their retirement funds were crashing, some more than 50 percent.

I had about a hundred emails from Abby's coworkers that I had been writing the market letters to for the last several years. Massive changes were also coming to their retirement account options, and they had a lot of questions. There were so many that Abby's employer issued a freeze up warning to her about the heavy e-mail activity. I must have had at least fifty people tell me this meant working for several additional years to over-come. They are probably right. I felt terrible for them. I still do. It means nothing to have made a great market call only to have had nobody listen that you wrote it for.

I tried to block the anxiety out, but I couldn't, even though I knew better than to let this affect me like it was. I still hadn't been able to grieve over my sister yet. But I knew these friends and associates were hurting—some hurting pretty badly. As tough as I try and have tried to act, I'm really not able to block out others' pain that I care about one bit.

I know too well what it feels like.

●　●

Cedar Fever season in Austin can be the toughest time in the world on allergy sufferers. It starts about mid-December and usually ends in mid-February. The allergy symp-toms alone can be so severe as to put people in the hospital every year for it.

Of course, the holiday time of the year is the most stressful on many of us, perhaps even more so with the sick and diseased. We had large annual Christmas celebrations at our home that took days to prepare for. I was using the Cedar Fever as an easy denial and excuse tool, but the reality was the added anxiety of the holiday's demands had begun over the past few years to substantially weaken my immune system in coincidental timing with the allergy season, causing these infections to come on time like the French rail system.

I wound up getting my usual infection, right on schedule, around Christmas. It had been that way every year since the car wreck. Only this time, it was different, more flulike in feeling and leaving me very weak. Seemed worse than any infection I'd had to date.

With good reason, it was my thyroid that was severely infected this time, not my sinuses. After fifty-one years of disease, misunderstanding, neglect, denial, hiding, and justification, my thyroid had become the weakest point of my body, not my sinuses like usual. And white blood cells, our body's infection fighters, were attacking my thyroid gland like an old enemy.

But I didn't know it. I was used to being sick and feeling bad all the time by now anyway.

*Just not this bad*, I thought, but, of course, would never admit.

*And I always get these infections every year. Terrific!* Routine medical self-diagnosis by an egomaniac who is past denial and doesn't even have a college degree. I continued the same lying charade with every family member and friend I had when they questioned me about my health and worsening appearance over the past few weeks. "This is nothing," I said, "just routine allergies. No problem." I continued to deny.

Right up until I lost my voice again, for the second time that month.

●  ●

I had a warning about how bad things were getting on Monday, December 29, 2008. I had what I originally thought was another panic attack, just a little worse than those before. This should have been, and was, the warning to get me to the hospital and get Doc Mike involved. But I shoved it down again, although I was just barely holding on by my fingernails. Abby was exhausted from her end-of-year business travel and hosting of the annual Christmas celebration we held at our home. I managed to send her to bed early so I could hide what was happening to me. It took three-quarters of a bottle of XO Brandy plus three narcotic-based pain pills to put me to sleep for about three hours that night.

Those were the last hours of sleep I would get until Friday night, January 2, 2009.

It happened early in the evening, and at first I thought I was having a heart attack. I didn't feel like I could breathe, and my heart rate was way too fast. But after thinking it through a few minutes, with Abby's fourteen years of experience in sales of medical equipment to the cardiology field to help me, we knew it wasn't a heart attack. The proper symptoms just weren't happening.

But I should have gone to the hospital anyway. A big hospital in Austin.

Instead, I looked my symptoms up on the Internet and assured myself it must be just another panic attack lasting longer than normal. The only problem was that panic attacks are only supposed to last a few minutes. My attack had been going on for several hours now, with no letup in sight.

It was no panic attack. And when would I ever learn to stop diagnosing myself?

If this happens to you, you must go to the hospital immediately without delay, and to a major hospital, even if it means a long drive to a larger city. You may not be able to be diagnosed at smaller hospitals because they won't have the necessary blood-testing instrument to diagnose an adrenal problem. It's very expensive and relatively rare equipment.

What was really happening to me, I learned later from Doc Mike, was that I had begun to "leak" adrenaline fluid throughout my entire body. My thyroid was starting to fight back against the infection and the attacking white blood cells.

I got up and went to the office on Tuesday, December 30, but could not work and left at noon. I was beginning to have the worst clammy hands and temperature control problems of my life. My feet were so cold Abby could hardly touch them, so we put heating pads on them while I was sweating profusely around the forehead and under my arms.

I could not hide the problem on Tuesday night. It got so bad for a few moments it flattened me against the wall of our home and I was unable to move or speak. This is the syndrome incident I have talked about earlier with my old foreman, Don. When your thyroid is "bursting," "leaking," or out of control, you will literally freeze up. You cannot walk properly or speak clearly. Combat veterans have a term that is similar to how we look. It's called "the thousand yard stare."

Abby almost went ballistic, but I kept her from calling for the ambulance. In our rural area, it would have been better to drive ourselves rather than wait on them. I kept assuring her I would be better; this was just a reaction to the "Cedar Fever" allergies that always came this time of year.

I got myself back together after a bit, but I was far from okay. I quickly killed the rest—over half of a bottle of fine single malt Scotch I had picked up with Dan north of Carnoustie on our golf trip to Scotland the previous March. That helped settle me down enough to get Abby relaxed with the way I looked and go to bed. I went to bed with her but did not sleep and crawled out around 1 a.m.

I was afraid I was losing my mind.

But this wasn't a mental problem. It was a serious, now life-threatening, medical problem.

The same one I had been lying, covering up, and hiding from all my life. Coming right back at me full speed.

And things were coming to a head.

      •     ●

I went to work on the Internet all Tuesday night, trying to figure out what was wrong with me. I knew I had to get to Doc Mike. This was the worst I had been in my life, but I knew he would not be there on New Year's Eve and closed on New Year's Day itself. I thought for sure I could tough it out until he got to his office the following Monday.

But I couldn't.

By Wednesday morning, New Year's Eve, I had begun leaking so badly I was ruining my clothing around the neck. My sweating was so full of adrenal fluid that it was causing the dye to come right out of my shirts.

A new problem began that I have never experienced before or since. I began to get quite clumsy, knocking things over constantly, dropping things, unable to walk or move in a normal fashion. I had never been like this, and it only added to the anxiety that was almost beyond what I could handle as it was. But it's a very serious sign—about the last one you may ever get in your life if you have a diseased thyroid gland.

Unless you're given the gift of a miracle, or miracles, like I was.

My infected and diseased thyroid gland that was being attacked by my own body's white blood cells had decided to fight back with everything it had. Everything.

The medical term is *thyroid storm.* If you look it up, it is simply listed as "fatal." The best statistic I can find out about a thyroid storm is that it is 90-percent fatal. Usually the survivors are always under the age of ten years old. It appears almost all of the rest die of acute myocardial infarction, a very sudden fatal heart attack. Their hearts just "blow up" due to the massive adrenaline in their bodies from the thyroid storm of adrenaline they've suffered.

I don't know the reason, but I hope to learn someday why I was spared.

But unbelievably, the miracles weren't over—yet.

I was already coming down from the adrenal levels I'd been to by Friday morning. I know this, even though I don't have the T-4 blood counts to give you to prove it. I know my body, and I know I was much lower in adrenal level. Even so, I ruined the shirt from that day's visit to Doc Mike's office. As expected, he was gone for the holiday, but I knew I couldn't wait any longer. He has the best staff you could find anywhere in town anyway, far better than an emergency room.

I had done so much research on the Internet during this time; I kept coming across "hyperthyroidism" as a very suspect problem. I took a symptoms list off the Internet and filled it out to take with me. It looked like I was a poster case.

The physician assistant who interviewed me was surprised but pleased at the proactive nature of my completing the symptoms list and did admit, despite the obvious stresses I had been under, that this could be a thyroid problem. Right about then, I began the "thyroid blush" all over my body. I pulled my shirt up to show her. I was bursting again at the time, going red all over, and I remember her look changed. She said, "This really does look like a thyroid problem. We need to run the t panels to check you out." I agreed. I had read this was one way to determine if a thyroid problem existed using a simple blood draw.

Doc Mike's lab ran the complex blood count, or CBC as it's commonly referred to, and then immediately sent the blood out for the complex adrenal analysis to a specialized lab. Doc Mike's office had found extremely high numbers of leukocytes in my blood—the white blood cell infection fighters that were attacking my thyroid at that very moment. I told the attending PA not to worry about those; it was common for me this time of year to have mild infection due to the Cedar. She took my word for it. I sure sounded like I knew what I was talking about. She then prescribed a sleeping aid and "something to just calm your thyroid … a very small dosage of Xanax." This was the *exact* course of treatment that was necessary.

I desperately needed the sleeping pills but would never tell her I wouldn't take the Xanax if my life depended on it (which it did). I had heard about Xanax before. I just smiled and agreed to her recommendations, and we left on Friday midday.

I was too afraid of Xanax. This was too much like my mom. I could hold out on those I was sure.

But ultimately, I couldn't.

I got both prescriptions filled but only took the sleeping pills at early bedtime. I was totally fatigued by now, like I had run a marathon, but had managed to eat a little food. It was the first food since Monday.

I took three of the sleeping pills, had some wine, and knocked myself out for a few hours.

●  ●

I awoke on Saturday morning to two serious problems. The first was a colored discharge from my sinuses that had indicated serious bacterial infection in the past, and two, I was beginning to have the heart attack feelings again. Abby was not up yet; it was about 5 a.m.

I was going to make Abby a surprise breakfast but could not walk straight to the kitchen and dropped the first pan I pulled off our overhead rack. I couldn't cook. I really couldn't stand. I went into the living room and went into the thousand yard stare. In retrospect, I know I began hallucinating. I don't know for exactly how long.

I also felt another storm was coming, and I was completely terrified.

I finished what was left of the XO Cognac a little before 6 a.m. It wasn't enough to help much, but it helped some. I just mentally refused to drink anymore. I could make it until 8 a.m.

when Doc Mike's office opened. This obviously was a bad infection; I could hardly breathe all morning. I had nearly lost my voice again for the third time in three weeks and had a very bad sore throat.

Abby woke up a little after 6 a.m., and when she saw me, she hit the roof. She called the small hospital in our county to determine if they had the lab capability to run a thyroid panel STAT. They admitted, after about twenty minutes of very defensive argument with her about their abilities, that they did not have the instrument to determine my adrenal level.

Obviously, not much help there.

Forget that; call Doc Mike's office and get an antibiotic for the infection. That will cool the thyroid down. Remember, all this time, I had the prescription right in my hand for the Xanax they had prescribed—the exact proper treatment in the smallest sized dosage level. I just wouldn't take it.

Mike was not in, and I was not going to call his mobile on his day off, but the physicians at his office refused to prescribe a strong antibiotic over the phone not only to "Doc Mike's buddy" patient but also because they didn't know me and I had just refused a similar prescription the day before. It was my fault I did not take the antibiotic prescription with me, by diagnosing myself, but even worse, I would not take the most important part of the medication prescribed—the Xanax—to cool off the thyroid. That was the biggest problem I had. The solution was in my hands, but I was far too afraid to use it.

I wouldn't wind up like my mom had. Never! Not "tranquilized" for my life, and with Xanax, I'd be addicted too. I would *not* do that. I would *die* first.

So I nearly did.

B y noon, we were on our way to the small hospital. I knew the doctors there could not properly determine much of my problem, but I could at least get an antibiotic. That should help until I could just tough this out.

But you simply can't tough out a diseased and infected gland. If not treated, the gland, or more likely, both of you will die.

I was afraid I *was* dying, inside; it felt like I was near the end.

I had demanded to drive. I was wild eyed, in another thyroidic skin blush of purple and red body color, all in tandem with a huge adrenal burst, which made it difficult for me to speak clearly and maintain my balance. Abby, against her better judgment, knew she could not argue with me. There also didn't appear to be time for it. Quickly, I had the car up to over one hundred miles per hour. On a two-lane country road. Abby was terrified, but she could tell things were very, very bad by now.

That's when the last of the miracles happened.

On a holiday weekend Saturday, during lunchtime, right in the middle of Doc Mike's bowl game he was watching, he just got up and decided to go to his office.

He can't give me a reason he did that to this day. Out of the blue? Do you think so?

That action, along with what he did when he got to his office, saved my life.

He heard what had happened with Abby's frantic calls when he got in and immediately called my house first, but we were already on our way to the hospital by then. So he called my mobile. I could hardly speak, so Abby took the phone and answered. She told him we were going to the small hospital in our county. He said, "Forget it. He may die there. Put him on the phone."

Abby handed me the phone, and Doc Mike said, "Stop the car and turn around. They can't help you there" (meaning the hospital). Then he asked me if I had taken my Xanax. I didn't lie. I didn't have the energy and was totally broken down. I told him, "No, Mike. I'm afraid to take them!" I had stopped the car on the shoulder by now.

He spoke to me in a manner and tone he had never used with me in our whole relationship. He told me in a very, very hard and strong manner that belies this gentle healer's nature and actually growled at me, "This is where you're going to get in trouble and die. This is a baby aspirin-sized dose; we both know it won't cure you. It's a Band-Aid, and with a Band-Aid you'll heal twice as fast. Without one, you probably don't have a chance with or without the antibiotic. I will take you down off this when it's time. Get in the passenger seat, swallow the pill, go home, and I will call you."

There was nothing left to do then. This was ugly, but I knew it as the truth. I couldn't make it anymore without some help. I swallowed a full tablet and moved to the passenger seat. It took about thirty minutes to get back home. By then, I was already rapidly improving. It turned out as Doc Mike had suspected. I did have a massive infection in my thyroid gland as well, so he called in a combat strength antibiotic that also began to work immediately. By the next morning, I was a different man.

And I was alive. My thyroid gland may not live much longer. But I believe I will.

⬤　⬤

The drug therapy has been and currently is working quite well for me. Calming my thyroid gland down has resulted in a much healthier and happier person than I've been in years. I have not had to come up to the prescribed dosage but once or twice in the entire time I've been "clinically addicted" to Xanax. Doc Mike wants me to manage my drug usage at the lowest possible level I can tolerate without too much discomfort. To assist in keeping the medication use down, I've added a great deal of exercise and dietary discipline to my lifestyle. This has resulted in many positive side effects, is not very expensive, and will almost surely help me live both a longer and better life.

Doc Mike and I also both know that during especially stressful times at work, when I'm traveling long distances, or sometimes just because the thyroid is leaking extra, I need to adjust the dosage slightly up. It becomes trial and error, and I've learned to err on the safe side depending upon the situation. There's been a great side benefit to this; I've had to prioritize my anger or be forced to take more medication. I dislike taking any additional medication beyond the minimum amount I must have, as I feel it slows me down too much. In any case, it's turned into an unexpected positive side effect that's resulted in a terrific natural time-out behavior improvement benefiting not only every relationship I have but also my overall health.

It's believed I'm either in the late stages of Hashimoto's syndrome or the last stages of Graves disease. I say believed because there is no definitive positive test for either disease. The diagnosis must be perceived by the physician(s) as the most likely of several outcomes from congenital thyroid tumors combined with adrenaline leakage. Hashimoto's thyroid disease is where the body's own immune system attacks and eventually destroys the thyroid gland. Graves disease (much more common in women) is another form of attacked and dying thyroid gland, or one that will probably go completely dysfunctional or inactive before the sufferer's body would die of other causes.

It could also be that my thyroid gland is just worn out from the leakage and overactivity for more than fifty-one years. There's not a doctor anywhere, of any specialty, who can tell me for sure. It's also believed my current disease situation is one that's ripe for developing into cancer, so I'm blood-tested very regularly for any unusual blood cell counts that can be a tipoff that cancer may have developed in my thyroid gland.

A good imagery of my current disease situation is one like

a sputtering lawnmower running out of gasoline while you're mowing. For sure it's going to quit in a minute or so, but you're desperate to get the last strip of lawn done.

I've got two options if I can stay cancer free. Stay on the drug therapy, currently Xanax, rotating similar drugs each a year at a time until either the gland gives up or I give up due to the ever-growing discomforts of adrenaline leakage. The alternative is to have the thyroid gland removed entirely and go on adrenaline substitutes for the rest of my life. Without the drugs, I doubt I could last a week; I would most likely have a heart attack and/or another thyroid storm, as the gland would soon begin to leak out of control.

With adrenaline leakage, it's a bit different than with a plumbing leak around your sink. In my lifetime of experiences, sometimes your gland can work just fine; much of the time it can't. This will in turn create "good" metabolic periods, where I can digest and get proper nutrition out of my food, relax, be outgoing and jovial, a much happier period, and "bad" metabolic periods, where I shouldn't eat much other than fruit or dried fruit, have a lot of trouble with irritability, anxiety, nausea, and a lessened ability to concentrate and perform at a high level as well as the many other symptoms you've already read about.

The more severe the leakage, the less "good" periods and the more and longer the "bad" periods. Combine growing adrenaline leakage with the natural process of the metabolic system slowing, and you have a recipe for obesity. In my opinion, the international spread of obesity isn't just because we're building more McDonald's restaurants around the world. I believe without a doubt we're handing thyroid disease down to our children every day of the week. And doing it unknowingly.

This is the biggest fear of thyroid disease I have now. An epidemic occurring.

Understanding then treating what's wrong with me has given me new hope in life and ended a great deal of fear I've felt for years. But a new uneasiness is taking its place. A strong suspicion we have a growing epidemic around the world of mis-diagnosed and undiagnosed thyroid disease.

In 1995 the Colorado Thyroid Disease Prevalence Study conducted a random, cross sectional study in a statewide health fair to look for both elevated and decreased TSH levels (the measures of adrenaline and thyroid activity). They tell a disturbing tale fourteen years ago. The incidence then of elevated levels of TSH was 9.5%, and the incidence of decreased TSH levels was 2.2%. That totaled almost 12% of the population with TSH levels out of range. Another phrase for clinical disease state.

The thyroid cancer disease statistics are worse. Since 1990, cancer statistics show the overall thyroid cancer incidence across all ages in the US has been subject to an annual increase of 1.4%. This is far more than statistically significant, it's alarming, but the facts went almost unpublicized except in specific scientific circles. The increase of cancer was highest among females at an increase of 1.6% per year, and it's worth noting that between 1975 and 1996 the incidence of thyroid cancer rose 42.1% in the US. In 1996, the incidence of thyroid cancer was 8% per 100,000 people.

With children, if you can believe it, the numbers were even more disturbing. The National Cancer Institute reported after the Colorado study that the most prevalent carcinomas (cancerous tumors) in US children and adolescents younger than twenty years of age was thyroid carcinoma at 35.5% of all children's cancers. Some shocking news that may be as old as your child or grandchild.

What about today? It's much worse, almost unimaginable. The National Cancer Institute reports that as of 2007, the incidence rate of thyroid cancer has grown from 8% per 100,000 in 1996 to 9.6% per 100,000 in 2007. This is in people of all ages and races. A full 20% increase in only eleven years, on the heels of a 42% increase in twenty-one years. The shocking statistics are in real numbers that 1 in 119 men and women alive today will be diagnosed with cancer of the thyroid in their lifetime. That's almost 1% of every single man, woman, and child in our country with thyroid cancer, not just thyroid disease! These are the facts, and in my opinion, they represent an epidemic bordering on the out of control.

What's causing it? There is no accepted clinical certainty yet. The gland is still too misunderstood and the research too limited (low awareness and funding plus a highly complex problem) for definitive answers that specifically address the why with factual medical science authority. There's a growing suspicion in the research community spearheaded by the New Zealand Government that soy products used in infancy may be a big factor. Others, especially research scientists from the UK and the US, feel that genetics and heredity are combining to grow the disease to these extreme proportions. It will take a good bit more detailed study to find out the answers. That means time.

Until then, sufferers have to be treated and deal with (not hide or hide from) the fact that we don't understand the scientific reasons for why we're anxious, and our doctors don't either.

All of us who have thyroid disease have an important job to do. Awareness. Many of us have hidden out, alone and in silence for a long time about our disease. There are many reasons for that hiding, but I believe it's got to stop. All it appears that staying silent has accomplished is to have kept the disease from reaching the awareness stage that leads to more effective treatments and eventual cures. Look at the cycle of defeated diseases over the past twenty-five years or so. The pattern is obvious. Raise awareness first, leading to the most important and crucial step of raising money. When money is raised, research begins or grows in intensity. Intense research results in improved treatment(s) and sometimes a cure. I feel thyroid disease is very low in our country's awareness, especially in light of the huge numbers of those that are suffering. So all of us, whether you're the one who is diseased or the friend/loved one/family member of a sufferer, there's an obvious need for focus on raising awareness about the disease and how it's growing. It's probably doubtful a cure will come in most of our lifetimes, but with science you never know, and for sure we could help generate one for those that follow.

One thing we do know after several years of research (or just a few pages of this book). Deny anxiety and/or metabolic disorders that are occurring in your body, for any period of time, and you're most likely going to wind up in big trouble. Or worse.

# The End of the Charade

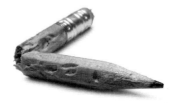

I'm close to the end of my story now, but I don't feel I'm close to the end of my life by any stretch. I hope it's more obvious now the story wasn't meant as an autobiography at all. It really was one man's story of how not to handle a lifelong disease. I've done an awful lot of things wrong over the years—so wrong I felt I had to write about it so maybe others wouldn't do the same.

I don't want you to do the same or for someone you care about to either.

That would make, in my mind, what I've done and was doing a real wasted life.

Happiness and peace for me is in the understanding. I understand my thyroid gland may be dying, but I'm not. I hope I don't face the decision of thyroid removal surgery or cancer very soon, but I'll face it differently and understand it better than ever before—of that I'm sure.

I've also learned I don't have any allergies at all. Zero. None. I do have some sinus disease related to being "thyroid hot" for fifty-one years, but that's not fatal either. Several other issues are already gone away or vastly improved now that I'm in the correct treatment. Symptoms like anxiety, depression, anger, denial, justification, arthritis, and most of the skin disorders aren't history, but they're not running my life like they used to.

I'm not moody much anymore either. I've learned I'm a calmer person than I ever thought I was. Some of the things I've found out have been a bit shocking to be honest.

I've also learned I'm not Superman, and I don't expect myself to be him anymore. In all honesty, right now, I wouldn't even qualify as Underdog.

So I've gone around to every one of my most important friends and told them I have been hiding things and keeping things from them about my health, just like an alcoholic does in the twelve-step program. After those meetings, I felt more than just loved. Not one friend has turned away from me, even though I have lied to them for years.

I am *clinically diseased* and I'm in a *clinical addiction*. These are serious terms about serious issues we'll discuss at length later in this book, but from the point of view of a sufferer only. Not that of an MD. I don't diagnose myself anymore.

That's Doc Mike's job.

I'm too busy and not qualified for that. I've got a life to live now.

●  ●

Before I close this chapter, I have a few questions I want to ask those of you who have read some or all of this book and realize they may have a few problems or may be sick.

1. Do you have a doctor that sounds like Doc Mike? If not, you better be lucky. And you've got to get to work finding one. It may really mean your life.

2. Do you want to take the chances with your health I've taken, ultimately relying truly on miracles just to survive?

3. Do you think the behavior examples I've written truthfully about are the types of behavior you want to practice? Or for your children, parents, or friends to practice?

These are pretty simple questions, but if the answer to any of them is "No," then the real question becomes, "What are you going to do about it?"

There are some thoughts in the final chapter about just exactly what you can do about it. But it's not for me to preach to you or anybody else about facing health issues and fears by ending denial. I've been far too guilty of this behavior for far too long now. You were smart enough and honest enough about things to read this book.

You're smart enough and honest enough to get a proper diagnosis and treatment.

It's now just a matter of whether you'll face up to it or not.

And if you'll do it, you *will* ultimately find out the answer to, "Why am I anxious?"

# A Note to Caregivers

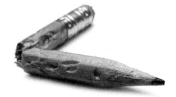

For Loved Ones, Friends, Family, and Guardian Angels of Those Who Are Sick with Anxiety-Type Disorders.

You're reading this book because you suspect someone you love or care about may be sick with some of the symptoms you've read about inside, and to follow, in this book.

You are potentially the most important person in your friend's or loved one's life.

Especially right now. At this very moment.

There are many reasons why your friend isn't being treated or getting better. You've read about most of the mistakes one could possibly make inside already. But for some, it may be for financial reasons they're not going to the doctor. They can't afford it, they think. But have they talked to their family doctor about a payment plan? You might ask them, or better yet, help them when they have that talk with either their doctor or their doctor's business manager. Very, very few doctors, especially general practice healers, won't work with your friend on a payment plan, even if your friend has no insurance. These doctors can many times also get your friend on proper drug treatment at little or no cost as well through their referral to many drug companies' financial assistance programs.

So financial reasons are basically just another excuse, one I was lucky enough to never have had to use. But you can bet if

I'd had reason to, I probably would have used it as well. I've used every other excuse I could think of. And I'm not proud of it.

The excuses also may be because your friend, who appears to have a lot of suspicious symptoms to you, may be in hiding or in denial like I've talked about I was in for so long. A great many of us are doing this, I believe. And we get sensitive about it and won't talk to you honestly regarding it. At least many times we won't until we're broken all the way down, and by then, it may be too late for us.

You may be rebuffed at first when you approach your friend, even treated angrily and possibly abusively. But if that happens, you've got to know you've hit a home run. We're angry because you've found us out, not because you care! And believe me, that's terrifying to us. You've hit us hard with your caring. We work awfully hard at our hiding, wasting hours a day of our time along with tons of effort. We may try to avoid you after that for a while. But don't fall for that; expect it! It's an act! An act of fear mostly.

So then you have to show a lot of casual interest in our health over time in order to gain our trust. This takes an awful lot of work and can be quite frustrating. Just remember, eventually, after you've done this for a while, almost all of us will let slip what we know the main problem is. The big question then becomes, "Will you be listening?" And I guess, more importantly, what will you do about it?

This is a very important decision. One of the most important decisions you may make in your entire life. And it may affect your own life forever.

So before you make a decision to not get involved or say something to yourself like, "I just can't help them right now with all I've got going on already," think about it one more time.

You already have the suspicion, and it's probably accurate. Remember, you were smart enough to read the book, so you're more than smart enough to be the difference.

A difference in a human life.

Whatever your decision may be, would you consider just another moment right now about what that decision is really all about? Being the difference in a human's life is what it's about! It's just staggering how important you can be—life-changing important.

Believe me. I know for a fact how crucial you are. I wouldn't be alive today without my difference makers. We need you desperately. Please don't give up on us.

## Common symptoms of thyroid, autoimmune, and anxiety disorders. This is not an all-inclusive list. Use this personally.

| *Thyroid* | *Autoimmune* | *Anxiety* |
|---|---|---|
| Heart rate feels high | Low body temperature | Heart rate feels high |
| Heart rate palpitates | Elevated fever | Irritable |
| Shaky | Dizziness and/or vertigo | Shortness of breath |
| Nervous and tense | | Nervous and tense |
| Long-lasting anxiousness | Long-lasting anxiousness | Long-lasting anxiousness |
| Diarrhea | Bloating and constipation | Diarrhea |
| Frequent urination | Frequent urination | Frequent urination |
| Temperature control issues | Temperature control issues | Temperature control issues |
| Skin is very dry | Acne | |
| Bad dandruff | Skin rash | |
| Poor sleep | Insomnia | Poor sleep |
| Cannot stay asleep | Minimal exercise exhausts | Cannot stay asleep |
| Unexplained weight change | Feel hypoglycemic | Unexplained weight change |
| Heavy perspiration | Fragile skin | Heavy perspiration |
| Hands or mouth trembling | Bruise easily | Tremors and twitches |
| Panic attack | Panic attack | Panic attack |
| Weak muscles | Weak muscles | Muscle tension |
| Frozen/very sore shoulder | Swelling in feet | |
| Undiagnosed allergies | | |
| Mood changes easily | Mood changes easily | Mood changes easily |
| Depression | | Depression |
| Feeling worthless | | Feeling of impending doom |
| Difficulty concentrating | Difficulty concentrating | Difficulty concentrating |
| Difficulty learning | Loss of coordination | Difficulty learning |
| Forgetfulness | | Forgetfulness |
| Recurring sinus infections | Mouth and nose sores | Headaches |
| Other frequent infections | Eye infections | |
| Loss of sex drive | | Loss of sex drive |
| Eyes sensitive to light | Dry eyes | |
| Eyes sometimes bulge out | Loss of vision strength | |
| Excess tooth decay | | |
| Extreme fatigue | Extreme fatigue | Extreme fatigue |
| Loss of body hair | Hair is rough and coarse | |
| Loss of head hair | Bald patches on scalp | |
| Arthritis or joint pain | Arthritis or joint pain | |
| Clumsy behavior | Clumsy behavior | Feeling of being keyed up |
| Dry mouth w/dehydration | Dry mouth w/dehydration | |

You can see from this list how tough an exact and specific diagnosis can be and how these medical disorders mimic each other across the spectrum. Ferreting out the true medical problem is very, very challenging, even to the smartest of our physicians. Do not give up on any doctor you trust because the first treatments don't work out the way you hoped they would. It's going to take work on both the part of the sufferer, our friends, and loved ones, as well as our doctors, to finally get to the bottom of the problem.

It has seemed to help Doc Mike and his staff when I have been very proactive about what's going on with my health and my symptoms. For example, the completion of the thyroid symptoms list *before* I went to their offices. Any notes you can make about how you feel when symptoms get high and/or very bothersome to you are most helpful to them. Things like the last time you had a temperature control problem. Was it after an event at work, home, or school, or were you simply watching television or driving to work and you got clammy hands and cold feet? Do you have cold feet a lot? What time is it happening? Anything you can think of to note, especially *exactly* how you feel. These can be absolutely critical notes for a doctor to review. Please don't underestimate them or think you need to put them on a fancy form like the one in the back of the book. Make a note on an envelope, or anything in hand, right when it happens. You *will* help yourself by doing this.

But keep in mind you can only help yourself if you actually *go* to the doctor. It won't help to make all the notes in the world and not show them to a physician you can trust.

Believe me, I know. I've done this before. But not any longer. I don't want you to either.

● ●

## Notes about the symptoms list and physician letter that detach from the back of this book:

The letter is a generic request letter to your doctor. You do not have to take this with you to make a request of these services by any stretch. I've simply found it easier for me to make a list of what I want seen about and/or to talk about at my doctor's office, much like a very small grocery list. This letter is basically just that: a list of things you want done to help determine if you may have a problem with your thyroid.

There are more than the three requested blood tests and sonogram that can help pinpoint exact thyroid disease. But virtually every doctor will want at least these particular tests done. At least every doctor I've spoken to has. But keep in mind they may want additional testing that I've not spoken about. It is your job to ask questions about these tests, whatever they are, until you are comfortable with why they are testing you, for what, and you are sure it's relevant to the type of symptoms you have. If you have doubts, keep asking questions. If you still have doubts about extra testing other than that you've requested from the letter here, you may need to just say no or need to find a new general physician.

It may not be the easiest decision you'll ever make to change doctors, but when your health and the potential of life-threatening disease is involved, it may likely be one of the most important resolutions of your life. You'll have to act like it is, by being strong, committed to positive change and health improvement, and becoming the boss of your own health.

The three blood tests are first a complex blood analysis broken down into at least two parts, which starts with a CBC with Salts, or more simply put, a complex blood count with a look at body minerals. This part of the blood testing will do a very general overview of your blood to allow the doctor to know a great deal about what's going on with you in relation to normal body functions. The "salts" are to determine the mineral levels in your body, which, if too low in some cases, can easily mimic a lot of the same symptoms as thyroid disease.

The second blood test is much more complex T-3, T-4, free T-3, and free T-4, and TSH, or more commonly known as a "thyroid panel." You must be very careful here and speak to your doctor about what lab he/she uses for these tests. The instruments that run these tests vary widely in accuracy and capability, across the country. You only are interested in receiving tests that have *exact number readings*, not the type of machinery that can only give a result of "in range" or "out of range." In my opinion, these types of results can get you into a lot of trouble.

Where you are in the value of your panel reading is very important in my opinion. If you are toward the low end of the spectrum and you are having weight problems, some depression, low energy, a tough time concentrating, regardless of whether you are still "in range" as determined by an outside laboratory's equipment, you could still have a problem with your adrenaline, thyroid gland, or metabolic system. Keep it simple. Tell your doctor you want to see your exact thyroid test numbers, not a range report, and that you want to know if the laboratory instruments used were built after 2007. If they are, they'll be able to detect to the current day American Thyroid Association standards. If there is a problem with that or you're not getting complete answers that you understand fully, you're probably at the wrong doctor.

When your blood draw is being done, your doctor may have strong suspicions about things and ask for permission to run additional tests. Some I have had run that were very helpful to me were a complete vitamin panel. I've learned that many folks with thyroid problems have vitamin deficiencies, many times caused by either too much or too little adrenal fluid. I have a vitamin A deficiency we believe is linked to my disease. I have heard of others who had vitamin B, C, and E deficiencies. A vitamin panel is worth running and is not the most expensive of tests. It's known that serious vitamin A deficiency is a major contributor to skin problems. Why it's common in thyroid disease sufferers is not.

I have started a major vitamin supplement program after speaking at length about it with Doc Mike. With his whole-hearted blessings, I can report there is a positive effect. With me it's been with better energy, sex drive, and ability to work better and more productively. These improvements started even before my positive diagnosis because I began them before any testing was completed. Vitamins aren't cheap, but if they make you feel better in any way, in my opinion, they're more than worth it.

Another test I've done, mostly to rule out wrong diagnoses, which are obviously so easy to occur, is a detailed urine analysis. This will help your doctor rule out a lot of things that can mimic many of your symptoms and allow the focus of your diagnosis to sharpen even more.

The second request in the letter is critically important. You want to get a full color sonogram of your thyroid, which is a pain-less and quick process. You must see if polyps, tumors, nodules, or irregularities are on the surface of the gland and exactly what size they are, if any. During this sonogram, your physician may also look closely at several important arteries around the thyroid gland, which are going directly to the heart. They can measure the walls of these arteries with the sonogram and tell you if you are at risk for plaque buildup on the walls of your arteries and whether you appear to be at a higher risk than normal for hardening of the arteries and other heart problems before they happen. It is a critically important test for anyone who is involved in diagnosis of a thyroid problem. In my case, the final correct diagnosis came here.

The third blood test is if you and your physician are still con-cerned about your symptoms and thyroid, even though all pre-vious tests have come back negative or inconclusive. It's called "toleration testing." It's not a fun, inexpensive, or short test, but it may be critical to your future health at this time. It will involve multiple blood draws after your blood has been directly exposed to adrenaline, ephedrine, and caffeine. The results will tell you and your doctor a great deal about your health situation upon completion.

Just like tolerance to alcohol, people's tolerance to adrenaline is different. Obviously, caffeine too. Just look at the number of no or low caffeine drinks and coffees on the market today. In other words, your thyroid gland may be working just perfectly, putting out the exact amount of adrenaline at exactly the right times; your body just won't tolerate that adrenaline like some people you know who can only have a single glass of wine before they get a bit tipsy and sleepy, while others can drink the whole bottle and you could never tell it. It is the exact same principle.

After these tests, you and your doctor will almost surely know if you have a thyroid problem, and you may find out you have some other health issues to deal with too. You may find out you don't have a clinical thyroid problem but have a different type of autoimmune or metabolic issue due to the range of testing that's been completed that has disguised itself as a potential thyroid problem. In many, many cases, you will be on your way to a final and complete diagnosis. But more importantly, the final and correct treatment. That's the only thing that counts.

Procrastinating, denying, and waiting can be the mistake of your life, maybe the last mistake you'll ever make.

I can't tell you something like "Don't do this!" It's absurd. I'm already guilty of doing it for at least twenty-five years and probably more. Saying something like that only brands me as a hypocrite, and of the worst kind too. I can only show you how impossible your situation will ultimately become through my own mistakes, but only if you're one of those lucky enough to live through years of mistakes like I was.

I'll leave it to your opinion to decide whether this sounds like a good gamble to you or whether you or a close friend might need to see a doctor right away.

Like tomorrow.

●  ●

# Some common questions, with my responses based on my personal experiences, not proper medical training. Ultimately, your doctor will have the correct medical answer.

*Why is it you don't hear more about thyroid disease? The numbers of people afflicted seem to be a great deal larger than I possibly imagined.*

I think there are several reasons for this. First, you can live without your thyroid, so having your thyroid taken out has become accepted among the general public like having gall bladder removal or one kidney taken out. "You can live without it, so it must not be life-threatening" is an attitude you get from people who don't realize that so many heart attacks alone are caused by thyroid storms. It's quite difficult to determine post-mortem if the cause of death was excess adrenaline for a great deal of reasons, many of them technological. But when you hear phrases like, "He just dropped dead, right on the spot!" or you hear about men and women who have "worked themselves to death," this is highly suspicious of thyroid storm or disease. Especially when the cause of death is ruled a myocardial infarction. There are simply not that many things that can go wrong in your body, or your environment, to "blow your heart up" unless you've just completely ignored high blood pressure and/or coronary disease for many years, which is very rare in America. But excess adrenaline, even for just a few minutes, sure can do it.

The second reason I think you don't hear a lot about thyroid disease in particular is that it's not well understood yet. It is a very complex gland that performs or regulates a great many functions in the body. How it does many of those functions and regulations are being studied very aggressively today but are not fully understood. In addition, the clinical study of thyroid disease and the amount of money to put into its research is a mere fractional percentage of the kind of money that diseases like AIDS, muscular dystrophy, and cancer receive.

You also may be surprised to learn there is not a single US-based foundation for sufferers of thyroid disease. There is a strong organization in the American Thyroid Association, but that is a clinical study group comprised of research scientists we need to help us learn about the gland itself. It doesn't "help" the public directly; that's not its mission. I know this because Abby and I have researched it to death and as a result are founding one ourselves. There is one in Canada and in the UK but not here in the US. Not one dollar that we know of is given in the US to help people in financial difficulty get specific thyroid-disease testing or treatment. To someone like me, you can see where this is hard to live with. I now consider this a war, with the best weapon being awareness, followed by enough money to get some people tested who are in real need of medical help. The National Thyroid Foundation is where the royalties of this book are dedicated to.

The last of the thoughts on the lack of media attention and general awareness of the shockingly high incidence of thyroid disease is a great deal of misunderstanding about anxiety symptoms and what they may represent, especially in those of us older than forty years old. Many of us in that age group are typically "baby boomers" that grew up with a lot of misunderstanding of what anxiety was, what it's caused by, and that it's a medical problem, not a mental one. As you've read, this can be a deadly misunderstanding. Thyroid disease evidences itself almost always in anxiety-type symptoms because the thyroid is our anxiety and "fight or flight" organ. Simply put, you can have clinical depression or clinical anxiety problems with a perfectly functioning thyroid gland, but you cannot avoid having clinical anxiety and/or depression symptoms if you have thyroid disease.

● ●

*Are you always born with this disease, like a birth defect, or can you develop it as your life goes on? What gives?*

Both are believed true. I know, regardless of lack of scientific evidence, that my mother and my sister had thyroid disease, and there is clear clinical evidence of it among my nieces and nephews and their children. My mom was like me I believe—"hyperthyroid"—and I believe my sister, Marcia, was "hypothyroid." The American Thyroid Association's *belief* for lack of a better term is that thyroid disease is genetic in nature and passed down and across blood lines. I am quite sure of it myself, but it is not a medically accepted fact yet as I understand it in spring 2009.

You can develop the whole range of thyroid diseases as life goes on. Tumors and nodules are very common problems that develop, along with infection and irregular function issues of the gland. Your tolerance can change too, which can be extremely difficult to diagnose without the toleration testing discussed earlier.

● ●

*Does thyroid disease affect one group of people more than another? One sex or race or anything like that?*

I don't believe the whole truth is known as to that, but of the diagnosed clinical thyroid disease sufferers in America, more than 60 percent of those documented are women. I can't honestly say after reading extensively about this that this is truly statistically significant in my opinion. I question the statistics because of population differences between men and women,

women generally living longer than men to develop the disease, and the fact that women, I believe, are much more likely to stick with it and get diagnosed than men are. If you are a man and you believe you may have a thyroid problem, don't believe for a second that because this disease may, as of now, "statistically" hit more women than men and you don't need to be tested.

There appear to be many more diagnosed hypothyroid cases than hyperthyroid, at a statistically significant level, about 69% hypothyroid, as I understand it today. If you have suddenly started gaining weight and have many of the symptoms from the symptoms list, you really must have your thyroid tested and perhaps some additional metabolic testing as well. These can be the early signs of hypothyroid disease, hormonal imbalance, and several other life-threatening issues. In addition, the added weight can raise your blood pressure and increase your heart-disease-risk chances.

There do appear to be small differences in thyroid cancer incidence amongst gender of different races; statistics say thyroid cancer is attacking the white male almost twice as often as the black male and 30% more often than the Hispanic male. The stats are similar for women, with white women being the most likely of all groups of women to develop both thyroid disease and thyroid cancer. The statistical results are recognized and currently studied energetically in Canada, Australia, New Zealand, and the UK. But unfortunately, thyroid disease appears to be indiscriminate and global in nature. To put it simply, it can and will infect and potentially kill anybody, anywhere.

•  •

*I can't have thyroid disease, I'm not bald or going bald.*

According to research, losing head hair only occurs about 55% of the time. That's barely significant statistically and certainly no reason for anyone to believe they don't have thyroid disease if they have many of the other symptoms. For one thing, has there been hair loss on other parts of your body? Like on your back, arms, or legs? Has your hair changed color, gotten significantly grayer, or changed to a coarse or very dry condition? How about new or renewed dandruff and/or scalp sores? These are all symptoms of thyroid disease that can occur without any or very little head hair loss.

Suddenly seeing head hair loss? It could be a glandular or metabolic problem, but keep in mind that this happens frequently to men and women who don't have thyroid disease for a variety of reasons. In any case, don't trust old beliefs about thyroid disease going hand in hand with going bald. Those beliefs are not statistically true.

•  •

*I don't have a "Doc Mike," and/or I don't have a family doctor.*

This may be okay if you're twenty-one, but by the time you're thirty or so, if not before, you need a general physician, preferably one you feel is a healer.

I describe a "healer" as a stubborn woman or man in the general practice specialty of medicine who won't quit until they get to the bottom of it. You will hear phrases from them like, "Don't worry, Bill; we're going to find out what's going on," or "Sue, we're going to stick with this until we fix it." I've found these are the kinds of things these "bulldogs" say.

In most of the healers' practices in my experience, you don't pay before you are seen! Sound simple? It's not, especially nowadays. I also avoid places that are called "Institute" of something or "Center" of something. I have found my best doctors all my life were people who simply put their name on the door, and if they have their own lab, they call it a general practice clinic or something similar.

Friends and family are great places for referrals. But I am wary of doctors who continually refer you to another physician. The buck needs to stop somewhere. It's my thought that sometimes along the way, some doctors can and do cross the line over the business of medicine, just like any other professional can be money driven too.

Yes, I have had to "fire" doctors, just like I have had to fire staff, contractors, workers, etc. You are paying the bills, maybe along with the insurance company, but it's your health that's involved. If you aren't happy with what you're getting or have a bad or less than impressed feeling, keep it professional and impersonal, but move along. You're probably not going to get diagnosed and/or treated there anyway. A loss of confidence is definitely a signal it's over; get looking for another doctor right away.

Establishing any relationship is at least 50 percent your responsibility. You've seen what a liar and cover-up artist I've been with my doctor who's also a good friend—such a good friend that he was one of the people I talked about earlier in the book that I have had to apologize to. But I believe you won't get healed without a crisis in your life if you won't trust your general practice doctor with the whole ugly truth.

Trust me; they can handle it. They will have heard worse.

Remember, of course, in order to be successfully treated, you can't act like I've acted either. You actually have to *take* the medications your doctor's office prescribed for them to help you, not just get the prescription filled.

●  ●

*What is this Xanax you've talked about and things like clinical addiction? Sounds scary.*

Xanax, Librium, Valium, and several others are in the class of drugs known as *benzodiazepines*. They are actually among the most commonly prescribed depressant medications in the US. They are not classified as tranquilizers but as depressants, and they are a controlled substance in almost every civilized country in the world.

Not understanding that Xanax wasn't a tranquilizer, like my mom had taken with so little success, was a big misunderstanding on my part that almost cost me my life. It's taught me to get on the Internet and learn about any drug I've been newly prescribed.

Benzodiazepines are most commonly prescribed for clinical anxiety, but they exist to treat a wide variety of medical conditions, one of which is a "hot thyroid." Xanax in particular does this by affecting a key neurotransmitter in the brain, which will basically slow nerve impulses in your body. It is highly effective in fighting hyperthyroid symptoms.

I take a small dosage—in a known clinical addiction that I agreed to with Doc Mike before I started—to "cool off" my thyroid. This type of therapy is widely used for many of the thyroid diseases. In my case, we're hoping to lower the thyroid activity for a while to perhaps keep it alive longer, as well as keep me from the discomfort you get from excess adrenaline and the resulting anxiety. It is extremely effective for me at a surprisingly very low dosage level, usually around one milligram per day. I have yet to need more than two milligrams in a single day.

You can abuse and misuse these drugs. You cannot mix them heavily with alcohol, and until you know how you'll react to certain dosages, you must be careful with their use in routine situations. In other words, you've got to pay extremely careful attention to your usage. These drugs are a controlled substance for a very important reason. If taken in overdose amounts, they will definitely kill you.

There are side effects. With me personally, short-term memory has become a problem, but at the same time, one of the known side effects of Xanax in particular has been that long-term memory increases. It has helped me write this book in better detail than I would have ever thought possible and far better detail than my friends who are in the book can believe. I laugh about this every day with them and tell them, "I can't remember what happened fifteen minutes ago, but I can tell you exactly what golf score I shot fifteen years ago at such and such golf club." You've got to keep your sense of humor, but I find myself hoping I can remember where I put my mobile phone a lot!

I use my old-fashioned daily planner (I'm old. I haven't learned to use my mobile phone as well as I could for this, but most can) to track my usage. I note the time and amount, usually one-half milligram, and keep that for Doc Mike if he asks how it's going. He doesn't have to though; he knows I'm watching how much I'm taking like a stock chart. I know if the daily dosage I need begins to rise, I need to talk to him soon.

Am I worried about the addiction part? Not really, in all honesty. I quit smoking many years ago, and that was tough, but I did it, so anybody else can too. I accidentally developed a morphine addiction for a few days after the car wreck, but that was nothing really, and there were very few effects to deal with. But with Doc Mike's help, I know I can come down off this very slowly and without discomfort when the thyroid issue is resolved one way or the other. We've agreed on a year. We'll see what happens then.

●  ●

*What are some of the things I can do while I'm awaiting diagnosis? Are there simple things?*

In my opinion, definitely. Let's talk about each one that I've done that's helped.

a.  Cut down, or better yet, cut out, the caffeine. Yes, you will notice some mild side effects, probably due to caffeine withdrawal the first few days, but quickly you will notice less anxiety, better ability to think, and a more relaxed feeling. This means cutting out the chocolate too, which has killed me to do because I'm one of those people that really love chocolate. But I developed caffeine toxicity after my thyroid storm, and I couldn't drink a half a cup of decaf coffee if my life depended on it today. Doing this will make a change in your life regardless of your final medical diagnosis. I promise.

b.  Consider getting on some vitamin supplements, not just a multivitamin but specific vitamins like vitamin A, C, E, B-6, and zinc. Talk this over with your doctor on your first visit, and if they give the okay, try them, and see if your general health improves or not. If you don't feel they're helping you, you can always stop them; just don't expect them to be a "cure."

c.  You may have to adjust your diet substantially. I did. I have had to stay away from meat far more than I would like to, especially the big juicy New York strips I love. My body just won't metabolize heavy steaks properly, and it hasn't done so for a long time.

That's one of the reasons we can gain weight with thyroid problems. We're eating like an undiseased person, but our bodies can only metabolize much less, so the rest of the food gets stored, as fat usually. You can fight this off with a lot of vegetables and solid fruits like apples, pears, and most citrus. It will make it easier to lose weight as well. Talk this over with your doctor on your first visit, and see what opinion they have about it.

d. For me, exercise has been critical. I was unable to exercise right away after my storm for many reasons. But once I knew I could walk distances again, I got on our road and began to walk like my life depended upon it. It has done wonders for me. It has reduced my usage of Xanax, lowered my weight and blood pressure, and I feel better more days than not, especially after a good exercise day. This is another behavior that will help you, in my opinion, whatever your final diagnosis is. You don't need an expensive gym. I don't have one within fifteen miles of my home. You just need the okay from your doctor, a pair of comfortable walking shoes, and the desire to feel better. Then just get out on the road, put one foot in front of the other until you get a little tired, then turn around and go back. Try to do it a little longer the next time until you get to forty-five minutes or so. No, it's not rocket science, but I promise you it works.

I know this isn't earth-shattering advice. I'm sorry. I don't have any of that. I really wish I did. If there is any of that, I haven't found it, and Doc Mike hasn't told me about it either. This is just simple, commonsense, good health behavior that I've found really helps me. I'll leave it up to you. In your experience, has it been the "simple" things that have worked pretty well for you in all kinds of situations in your life, or not? All I ask is that you give it a try.

There's no need any longer for you or someone you love or care about to worry, "Why am I anxious?"

You *can* find the solution. The only thing you can't do is quit.

You're too important. After all, I wrote this book for you.

# Thyroid Disease Symptoms Checklist

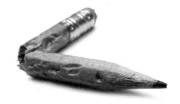

*(Feel free to tear out this list for your personal use)*

## *Your Heart*

- ☐ Heart rate feels high
- ☐ Heart seems to race
- ☐ Heart rate palpitates
- ☐ Shaky feelings
- ☐ Hands/mouth tremble

## *Your Digestion*

- ☐ Frequent diarrhea
- ☐ Frequent urination
- ☐ Watery, clear urine
- ☐ Recent weight gain
- ☐ Recent weight loss

## Your Sleep

- ☐ Cannot get to sleep
- ☐ Cannot stay asleep
- ☐ Poor sleep habits
- ☐ Wake up tired
- ☐ Avg. hours sleep

## Body Temperature

- ☐ Cold feet
- ☐ Cold intolerant
- ☐ Feel cold, others hot
- ☐ Feel hot, others cold
- ☐ Excess sweating
- ☐ Clammy hands
- ☐ Feel dehydrated
- ☐ Thick mucous

## Infections

- ☐ Allergies
- ☐ Sinus infections
- ☐ Frequent infections
- ☐ Swollen thyroid area
- ☐ Sore throat
- ☐ Lost voice
- ☐ Frequent nasal drip

## Your Moods

- ☐ Feeling shaky
- ☐ Frequent anxiety
- ☐ Nervous and tense
- ☐ Loss of sex drive
- ☐ Mood changes easy
- ☐ Depressed

☐ Worthless feelings
☐ Panic attack(s)

## Your Skin

☐ Very dry skin
☐ Frequent rashes
☐ Severe dandruff
☐ Loss of body hair
☐ Loss of head hair
☐ Loss of genital hair

## Your Vision

☐ Vision worsening
☐ Eyes sometimes bulge
☐ Eyes sensitive to light
☐ Night blindness

## Additional Symptoms

☐ Excess tooth decay
☐ Frozen/sore shoulder
☐ Difficulty learning
☐ Unable to concentrate
☐ Forgetfulness

## *Other Symptoms*

*Printed Name:*
*Birth date:*
*Signature:*
*Date:*

# *Request for Physician-Ordered Thyroid Testing*

Dear Physician,

This patient presents herself/himself with a symptoms list and requests you to help them learn if they have a thyroid problem or not. They have studied their health issues, and there is enough evidence in their belief to begin medical testing today.

First, please order detailed blood testing including a CBC with salts and a complete thyroid panel, including TSH. The patient needs actual readings of their T-3, T-4, free T-3, free T-4, and TSH, not a test that can only provide "in range" or "out of range" results. Please do not send blood samples to laboratories that cannot provide exact value results to both yourself and the patient. The patient will want a copy of the actual results.

Second, if those results come back near to out of range or out of range, according to the most recent guidelines of 2009 set forth by the American Thyroid Association, please consult with the patient on the order of a sonogram to study the gland for tumors, nodules, or irregularities of the gland itself. Please consider an order for a sonogram if you have professional suspicions of your own, irrespective of the patient's blood test results.

If the symptoms persist beyond the thirty-day mark without significant improvement and a final diagnosis has not been arrived at using both blood analysis and a sonogram, please consult with the patient the process of toleration testing and its cost and time involved. Please thoroughly discuss any referrals you are going to offer this patient and why you think this referral is vitally necessary and critically important to improving their health.

Please discuss dietary changes and thoughts on exercise that may be of use in this case. Please *stick with it* until this patient is not only fully and accurately diagnosed but in treatment and feeling better.

—Clay Ballentine
Chairman
National Thyroid Foundation

# listen|imagine|view|experience

## AUDIO BOOK DOWNLOAD INCLUDED WITH THIS BOOK!

In your hands you hold a complete digital entertainment package. In addition to the paper version, you receive a free download of the audio version of this book. Simply use the code listed below when visiting our website. Once downloaded to your computer, you can listen to the book through your computer's speakers, burn it to an audio CD or save the file to your portable music device (such as Apple's popular iPod) and listen on the go!

How to get your free audio book digital download:

1. Visit www.tatepublishing.com and click on the e|LIVE logo on the home page.

2. Enter the following coupon code:
   061e-f2af-8f73-a841-5858-6bc2-c679-6d4c

3. Download the audio book from your e|LIVE digital locker and begin enjoying your new digital entertainment package today!